Mary Elizabeth Hill Hanchey
and Erin McClain, eds.

# Though the Darkness Gather Round

Devotions about Infertility,
Miscarriage, and Infant Loss

# **Advance Praise for** *Though the Darkness Gather Round*

The number of those who have experienced infertility, miscarriage, or the death of a child are astoundingly high, yet all too often their tragic loss is met with silence. The voices of lament and hope in this wonderful book fill that void by retrieving a language of faith that speaks into the silence of grief and calls for gathering communities to surround one another in love.

—*Curtis W. Freeman*
*Research Professor of Theology, Director of the Baptist House of Studies*
*Duke University Divinity School*

Within a culture that deems some stories too painful to tell, these remembrances are raw, deep, and impassioned—delving into doubt, rage, grief, and the scars that never disappear. In other words, they are real stories of what it is to be human. This book will surely be a gift to anyone who has suffered the particular losses of infertility, miscarriage and infant loss, but just as surely it will be a gift to anyone who has ever struggled with love and its counterpart, loss.

—*LeDayne McLeese Polaski*
*Executive Director/Directora Ejecutiva, BPFNA—Bautistas por la Paz*

This gut-truthful, grace-laced collection of devotions stands in the gap between the larger people of God and our sisters and brothers who know fertility grief. For far too long, the church's silence and implied shame have held sway around these griefs and struggles. Here is a resource and gift to help us break the silence in a theologically honest and Biblically grounded way. Thanks be to God for the courage of all who brought this collection into being.

—*Alicia Davis Porterfield*
*Editor of* A Divine Duet: Ministry and Motherhood *and Pastor*

This devotional collection is a rich resource for those who travel on a trail of tears during the journey of faith. It is a gift because it shows how lament is a critical expression of faith even when tears may be one's food day and night. Through the tears of lament, this multivocal literary chorus sings a constant theme of hope, revealing how tears sow seeds of hope in the soil of faith. This hope has deep roots in a crucified God as it testifies of how God weeps with those who weep and bear their own cross of grief. This book may be tear-stained, but through the sad moisture of sorrow, every reader will hear the melody of hope, for "hope is a song in a weary throat."

—*Luke A. Powery*
*Dean of the Chapel, Associate Professor of the Practice of Homiletics*
*Duke University*

Smyth & Helwys Publishing, Inc.
6316 Peake Road
Macon, Georgia 31210-3960
1-800-747-3016
©2015 Mary Elizabeth Hill Hanchey and Erin McClain, eds.
All rights reserved.

*Library of Congress Cataloging-in-Publication Data*

Though the darkness gather round : devotions about infertility, miscarriage,
and infant loss / edited by Mary Elizabeth Hill Hanchey.
pages cm
Includes index.
ISBN 978-1-57312-811-7 (pbk. : alk. paper)
1. Mothers--Prayers and devotions. 2. Motherhood--Prayers and devotions.
3. Infertility--Prayers and devotions. 4. Miscarriage--Prayers and devotions.
5. Stillbirth--Prayers and devotions. 6. Newborn infants--Death--Prayers and devotions.
I. Hanchey, Mary Elizabeth Hill, 1970- editor.
BV4847.T49 2015
242'.4--dc23

2015013840

---

**Disclaimer of Liability**: With respect to statements of opinion or fact available in this work of nonfiction, Smyth & Helwys Publishing Inc. nor any of its employees, makes any warranty, express or implied, or assumes any legal liability or responsibility for the accuracy or completeness of any information disclosed, or represents that its use would not infringe privately-owned rights.

*This book, these sacred stories, are dedicated to
Chris Barrett
who now knows that his life on this side of heaven
will be much shorter than he had hoped.
And to his wife, Elise, and their children,
who must press on here.*

*Through loss and grief and suffering at various stages
and under varying circumstances, Elise and Chris
have attempted to love faithfully and bear witness with
as much courage and truthfulness as they could offer.*

*Thanks be to God.*

# Acknowledgments

On Ash Wednesday in 2013, Pam Durso, director of Baptist Women in Ministry, called me and said, "It is time for the book." I know it was Ash Wednesday because I remember talking to Pam while setting up for the service that would take place later that night—a service where we would remember together that we have come from dust and will return to dust, where we would mark even the smallest children among us with the cross, accepting the claim that Christ Jesus makes on our lives and our deaths.

Grief and hope and the following of Jesus into the desert during Lent were swirling in my very being as I stilled myself to listen. One never wants to miss a call to action from Pam. This book has come into being in no small part because of her insistence. And so, Pam, thank you for prompting me and for believing in this project.

This project has come into being as Project Pomegranate has come into being. I am grateful to Project Pomegranate co-founders, Erin McClain and Diane Paces-Wiles. We have worked tirelessly to build this ministry together, and we have built something to be proud of. I am especially grateful for the ways that Erin and Diane worked to shape this book of devotions. It is a powerful resource because of their wisdom and insight. Thank you to Erin, whose dining room table served as the sorting center and whose shuffling of these devotions on her table and in her mind led to the order and indexing that make this collection navigable and therefore helpful.

Thank you, also, to the team at Smyth & Helwys who have tended to so many publishing details. You turned our text into a really fantastic resource. Thank you for believing in this project!

The most important and profound thanks is owed to our writers. The Project Pomegranate team is grateful to so many who have shared their stories and their devotions with us. Thank you. These stories are poignant, powerful, and painful. Yet, with this collection of devotions, we sing together amid gathering darkness. We raise our voices to proclaim the things we know about God and the Son, Jesus, who sustain us. And we remember together that the "light shines in the darkness, and the darkness did not overcome it" (John 1:5).

—Mary Elizabeth Hill Hanchey

# Contents

| | | |
|---|---|---|
| *Foreword* | Laura Webb Smith | xi |
| *Introduction* | Mary Elizabeth Hill Hanchey | 1 |

## CRYING OUT IN THE WILDERNESS: WE WEEP, WE RANT

| | | |
|---|---|---|
| *Hannah Wept Much* | Diane Paces-Wiles | 5 |
| *Room to Grieve* | Kim Miller | 9 |
| *Because You Already Have the Scars* | Aleta Payne McClenney | 13 |
| *Grief Out of Season* | Christopher Ingram | 15 |
| *My God, My God, Why . . . ?* | Gail Powery | 19 |
| *The Mourning Is Never Far Off* | Blake Hart | 23 |
| *Grieving for and with Our Child* | Rebekah McLeod Hutto and William Joseph (B. J.) Hutto | 25 |
| *Throwing My Anger at God* | Jenny Barrier | 29 |
| *And then the Anger Came . . .* | Joanne Henley | 33 |
| *Beyond the Silence* | Chris Barrett | 35 |
| *When They Want Me to Speak* | Rick Jordan | 39 |
| *It's Not Okay* | Ryan R. Whitley | 43 |
| *Weary with My Moaning* | Sheree Jones | 47 |
| *Not Ready to Face the World* | Joy M. Freeman | 49 |
| *What a Friend . . .* | Erin K. McClain | 53 |
| *An Unlikely Prayer Partner* | Jennifer Andrews-Weckerly | 57 |
| *Absence* | Stephanie McLeskey | 61 |
| *God Never Left* | Rachel Whaley Doll | 65 |

| | | |
|---|---|---|
| *In the Wilderness* | Pam Durso | 67 |
| *Redemption in the Dark* | Rebekah McLeod Hutto | 71 |

## Light Shines in the Darkness: We Are Not Alone

| | | |
|---|---|---|
| *Grief Changes* | Mary Elizabeth Hill Hanchey | 77 |
| *Expecting* | Holly Jarrell-Marcinelli | 79 |
| *A Shared Hope* | Deborah Gaddis Reeves | 83 |
| *Deeply Marked* | Elise Erikson Barrett | 87 |
| *Where Does My Help Come From?* | Brittany Rasmussen Mackey | 91 |
| *Knowing You in My Heart* | Susan A. Joyce | 95 |
| *I Believe* | Katie Roscoe | 99 |
| *When I Was a Desolate Woman* | Anonymous | 103 |
| *When Suffering Gives Birth to Beauty* | Todd Maberry | 107 |
| *Resting My Eyes* | R. P. Fugarino | 111 |
| *The God Who Listens* | Sharon A. Buttry | 115 |
| *How Long?* | Jennifer Andrews-Weckerly | 119 |
| *My Limits Confronted Me* | R. P. Fugarino | 123 |
| *Movie People* | Brian Barrier | 127 |
| *Everything Happens* | Holly Jarrell-Marcinelli | 131 |
| *From Chaos to Stillness* | Joy M. Freeman | 135 |
| *That Much Faith* | Bekah Hart | 139 |
| *Barrenness and HOPE* | Pam Durso | 143 |
| *Life under Heaven Lives with What Is* | Mary McMillan Terry | 147 |
| *Shambles* | William Joseph (B. J.) Hutto | 151 |

| | |
|---|---|
| Index | 153 |

# Foreword

> How long, O LORD? Will you forget me forever?
> How long will you hide your face from me?
> How long must I bear pain in my soul,
> and have sorrow in my heart all day long? (Ps 13:1-2)

We all gathered at the German bakery on a Saturday morning, summoned by a friend we had in common. It turns out we all had something else in common. We had suffered infertility, miscarriage, or both. We told our stories. And we cried. We bemoaned the fact that some of us had gone through our struggles in silence. It was time to break the silence, so we shared chocolate croissants and talked. Even though I was no longer feeling the emotional drag of my miscarriage, I realized that to get past personal and communal shame, lots of healing work remained. My story became one strand in the web we formed that day, a web that runs through Project Pomegranate and the birthing of this book of devotions. Project Pomegranate provides spiritual resources to support those who have experienced infertility, pregnancy loss, or infant death, and to encourage this support in their faith communities. And my strand bears the story of waiting.

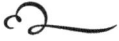

Our sweet neighbor, who also happened to be in the waiting room of our obstetrician's office that morning, excitedly inquired if we were expecting. His wife shushed him, and I caved at the awkwardness of the moment, looked away, and mumbled something about not feeling well. I wish I had looked them in the face and said, "I am scared we are losing the baby. Please keep us in your thoughts." I wish I had let them in on the hard waiting that we faced.

The ultrasound confirmed what the cramps were telling us, so we went home and waited.

> How long, O Lord, will the pain go on?
> When will the bleeding stop?
> How long, O Lord, will I feel ashamed, like I failed at this most basic act of humanity?
> God, give me grace to wait.

I am good at waiting. I had been on bed rest for more than six weeks during my first pregnancy, and I excelled at it. But this was different. Before, I had been resting for the noble cause of growing a person inside of me. Now, the wait was full of physical and emotional pain that had the almost certain result of ending my pregnancy. It was a wait I could not get behind. Would it be hours before I could resume life? Days? Weeks? When would the end actually come? Had it happened already?

After the initial waiting for the pregnancy to end, there was waiting to get pregnant again. Then waiting through each ripple and bump of pregnancy to see if everything would be okay on the other side.

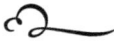

I wish that I had a profound conclusion to offer, perhaps an instruction manual for how to get through infertility, miscarriage, the loss of a child. A roadmap for the waiting. But all I can offer is my one thin strand. I weave it through the cramps and bleeding and waiting and disappointment and joy and hope of all the other strands. And I offer it to you with a prayer that God will give you grace to wait.

These devotions are for the waiting. They are for the long, dark nights. And the long, dark days. They are for those whose grief is personal—those who have suffered through infertility, miscarriage, and infant loss. They are also for family and friends and pastors and faith communities. This is an important resource. I pray that you will find devotions within this book that resonate with your strand in the web of life.

—Laura Webb Smith

**Laura Webb Smith** works, lives, and plays in Durham, North Carolina, where she enjoys adventures with her husband and two children, promotes positive environmental behaviors that protect our waterways, and worships at Watts Street Baptist Church. She is a friend of Project Pomegranate and a co-founder of the Hannah Ministry at Watts Street Baptist Church, which serves women and couples who have experienced pregnancy loss, infant loss, or infertility.

# Introduction

The title of this book, *Though the Darkness Gather Round*, may evoke for you the hopeful singing of its hymn, "How Can I Keep from Singing?" in the midst of some great grief. In singing the particular verse from which it comes, we make these claims:

> *What though my joys and comforts die?*
> *The Lord my Savior liveth;*
> *What though the darkness gather round!*
> *Songs in the night He giveth:*
> *No storm can shake my inmost calm*
> *While to that Rock I am clinging.*
> *Since love is Lord of heav'n and earth,*
> *How can I keep from singing?*

Many have sung this verse, and the others that come with it, weeping, sputtering out the words among deep heaves, claiming the songs we are given in the darkest night—even when singing them seems to be a gut-wrenching feat of madness. It has been my own prayer when no other words would come. It has accompanied me through funerals and long nights and hospital corridors. It has given me courage to cling tightly even as storms rage.

Much courage is required to weather the long grief of infertility and the sudden grief of miscarriage and infant loss. The storms that rage are frightening and overwhelming. And so this book, this collection of devotions by those who have lived through the gathering darkness, is much needed.

We have chosen forty devotions. "Forty" is a powerful number, evoking the forty weeks generally attributed to the full term of a pregnancy, the forty days and forty nights that Noah and his family huddled in the ark, the forty years the people of Israel wandered in the wilderness, the forty days Jesus spent in the desert, and the forty days that serve as the basis for the Christian season of Lent. Lent is forty days of darkness. Forty days of wandering and stumbling towards the life found in the resurrection.

It is our prayer that these devotions will be a resource to individuals who are wandering and stumbling through fertility grief—through infertility, miscarriage, and the loss of infants—and to the faith communities that walk beside them. May rage and encouragement and hope reside together. May we regain our singing voices, even if it is not for some time. So may it be.

—Mary Elizabeth Hill Hanchey

# Crying Out in the Wilderness: We Weep, We Rant

# Hannah Wept Much

## Diane Paces-Wiles

*And because the LORD had closed [Hannah's] womb, her rival [Peninnah] kept provoking her in order to irritate her. This went on year after year. Whenever Hannah went up to the house of the LORD, her rival provoked her till she wept and would not eat. Elkanah her husband would say to her, "Hannah, why are you weeping? Why don't you eat? Why are you downhearted? Don't I mean more to you than ten sons?" Once when they had finished eating and drinking in Shiloh, Hannah stood up. Now Eli the priest was sitting on a chair by the doorpost of the LORD's temple. In bitterness of soul, Hannah wept much and prayed to the LORD. And she made a vow, saying, "O LORD Almighty, if you will only look upon your servant's misery and remember me, and not forget your servant but give her a son, then I will give him to the LORD for all the days of his life, and no razor will ever be used on his head." As she kept on praying to the LORD, Eli observed her mouth. Hannah was praying in her heart, and her lips were moving but her voice was not heard. Eli thought she was drunk and said to her, "How long will you keep on getting drunk? Get rid of your wine." "Not so, my lord," Hannah replied, "I am a woman who is deeply troubled. I have not been drinking wine or beer; I was pouring out my soul to the LORD."* (1 Sam 1:6-15, NIV)

In many ways, Hannah has become the poster child for infertility—not merely because of what she suffered but also because her story brings together three things so often valued in Judeo-Christian tradition: faith in God, selfless sacrifice, and, ultimately, reward. Scan the Internet for sermons and devotionals about Hannah, and you'll see numerous reflections on her passionate prayer, her promise to give her child over to priesthood, and the fulfillment of her prayer in the birth of Samuel, a prophet heralding a new era. But for those dealing with infertility, this perspective on the story can feel empty. For some, no matter how fervently we pray and how many promises we make, the answer we want does not come.

Which is why, for me, the most significant line in the passage is this: "In bitterness of soul, Hannah wept much . . . ." Powerful. Unvarnished. Honest. Infertility is a lonely business, and this acknowledgment of the soul-crushing journey is critically important. Despite the prevalence in more than 12 percent of United States couples, infertility largely remains a taboo subject. In a recent national survey, 61 percent of infertile couples stated that they try to hide their fertility problems from family and friends. Rates of anxiety, depression, and other psychological issues among women with infertility are higher than for women who have cancer or heart disease. I suspect Hannah would not be surprised by these statistics.

Reflecting on the timeless truth of Hannah's story inspired me to rethink the passage for modern times. We may not be dealing with the unkindness of our husband's other wife or making burnt offerings to God, but the pain, the desperation, and the isolation are still very much the same.

For today's reader, Hannah's conflict with Peninnah speaks most clearly not to the rivalry between two wives but to the unsolicited comments women receive about their childbearing (or lack of). Imagine the scene: Peninnah's baby shower hosted, of course, by Hannah. Against a backdrop of pastel streamers and cuddly animals, Hannah is caught in the crossfire of well-meaning women. "You're next!" teases Peninnah's aunt. "Don't wait too long. You don't want to be an old mom!" chimes in a friend. "Oh, you know those smart career women," says Peninnah, giggling. "No time for babies!" At which point Hannah excuses herself to the bathroom, where she locks the door and sobs silently until it's time to cut the cake. During a struggle with infertility, the judgment of others can feel overwhelming. From the misguided remarks of friends to the parade of media images idealizing motherhood, we are told daily that we do not belong, we are lacking, we are less.

Even Elkanah, who loves Hannah deeply, stumbles in his attempts to comfort her. This, too, is familiar. Those who love us may encourage us to look on the bright side, saying in many ways, "Hannah, why are you weeping?"

"You have a nice husband and a good job!"

"Without children you can travel, go out to dinner, see friends whenever you want!"

"I love you. Isn't that enough?"

The truth? No. It isn't enough. However well intentioned, these comments dismiss real feelings of sorrow and pain. Infertility is grief. No spouse, friend, work, or fun can fill the hole of a desperately wanted child.

Hannah's promise to the Lord also stands the test of time. Who among us has not tried to strike a bargain with God? Surprisingly, the passage offers no words for Hannah's prayer, saying, "her lips were moving but her voice was not heard." In this omission the writer gives us a gift, inviting each person to fill in her own story. "What is your Hannah prayer?" the text asks us. "What words come at your darkest hour?" The Scripture does give us a sense of Hannah's state, noting that Eli the priest "thought she was drunk." If you have ever witnessed the ranting of an intoxicated person, you'll agree it's not a pretty scene. Emotions can be raw and primal, ugly and out of control. I may never have knelt at an altar at Shiloh, but I understand this desperation. Month after month of devastating disappointment left me crying in the diaper aisle at the grocery store or sent me into a rage with the arrival of a telltale pink or blue envelope announcing someone else's good news.

For sure, this passage offers hope and a reminder to trust in God. Yet there are times when keeping the faith is impossible in the midst of a long infertility struggle. When you feel weary and downhearted, it may be enough to find within the lines of this Scripture the permission to weep without judgment and the knowledge that you are not alone.

*Prayer*

Be with me, Lord
Here in the darkness,
In this place where hope is distant.
Choked by tears and rage,
I am lost.
Find me, Lord.
Hold me in my weariness
Until I can go on.
Amen.

**Diane Paces-Wiles** lives with her family in Durham, North Carolina, where she is a member of Watts Street Baptist Church and part of the Hannah Ministry planning team. She is a co-founder of Project Pomegranate. In 2015, Diane earned a master's degree in Social Work from UNC-Chapel Hill.

# Room to Grieve

## Kim Miller

> *They sat with him on the ground seven days and seven nights, and no one spoke a word to him, for they saw that his suffering was very great.* (Job 2:13)

A miscarriage is not a very tangible loss. To some, especially those who have not been through it, it is not thought of as much of a loss at all. It is a loss of someone who never got the chance to be. It is difficult to grieve the loss of something you have never seen or touched. It is even more difficult to support someone who is grieving that kind of loss. I think most people find it easier to dismiss the loss of something they cannot touch than to be present with the one who is grieving. It is a helpless feeling, not knowing what to do and being unsure of what to say. I can come alongside the helpless feeling, but that doesn't take away the pain of being on the receiving end of those who tried to help make it better.

After my miscarriage, I remember being told to "enjoy all these other children around here." The doctor said, "This just means everything is working right. You can get pregnant again right away." Others also encouraged us to "just have another baby and it will all be okay." And when we listened to that advice and our healthy daughter was born less than a year after our miscarriage, my own mother stood at my bedside and said, "Just think, if your first baby hadn't died, you wouldn't have this beautiful girl." Grieving was not an option.

I didn't have permission from those around me to grieve, and I did not give myself permission to grieve either. I was never able to see or hold my first baby, whom I miscarried at twelve weeks. I never got to hear a heartbeat or know for certain if it was a boy or girl. Everything and everyone around me sent me the message that it wasn't a big loss, and it must have been "for the best." So, as I had done many other times in my life, I stuffed the grief and pain into a box, shoved it away, and told myself, "I will deal with this later." Later was a long time in coming.

I went on to have three more children after the miscarriage, and suffered from severe post-partum depression after two of them. I believe my depression was as much a result of unresolved grief as of hormones or chemical imbalances. My husband and I rarely spoke of the child we lost. Our life was chaotic in more ways than one. I felt alone.

When we finally got settled, God began to show us our need for healing. Nine years after our baby died, my husband and I began to talk about our grief and loss, and we took action to acknowledge it. We believed that our baby was a boy, and we finally gave him a name, Selah Josiah. Selah is my favorite word from Psalms, often interpreted to mean, "to pause and reflect." Josiah is a name from the Old Testament that can be translated "YHWH saves" or "YHWH heals." We shared how we disappointed and hurt one another by not acknowledging the loss in the past. With the help of a counselor, we worked through the painful memories. We honored our baby with readings and prayers and shed tears we had long held back.

Many who have found themselves in deep grief like ours look to the biblical story of Job. Job was a righteous man who suffered great loss and whose friends gathered to offer their support. When they first arrived, they sat for seven days without speaking a word! It was the most profound and helpful thing they could do. In that silence they were doing nothing; they were simply being. They created a space for Job's grief.

This creation of space is a significant ministry to those who have lost pregnancies and children. The best way to support someone going through a loss is to simply be with that person. Being is harder than doing: my experience as a chaplain has taught me that. But sitting and listening is far more helpful than looking for the "right" words to say.

Furthermore, there is no timeline on grief, and grief will always leave a scar. It can be expressed immediately, or years later, and there is no "right" or "wrong" way to grieve. Don't be afraid of it. Don't be ashamed of it. Allow it to come. In my own story, I cannot sing verse 2 of "Because He Lives" without a tear. The grief always comes then. And this is the reality: my children who lived did not replace the one who died. But it is also true that making room for grief allowed me more room for joy.

*Prayer*

Most Gracious God,

It is not easy to grieve the loss of something that I have never been allowed to touch, and others around me often do not understand. However, I know that You are a God who is with me, even in grief. Help me to make room to grieve and not to be ashamed of it. Only in feeling this loss can I learn to make room for joy again when I am ready.

In Your Holy Name,

Amen

**Kim Miller** is a minister serving alongside her husband at Richfield Baptist Church in Richfield, North Carolina. She has recently completed her first chaplaincy internship and will soon start a second at Carolina Medical Center in Charlotte, working toward becoming a board-certified chaplain. Both Kim and her husband, Brian, graduated from Campbell University Divinity School with a Master of Divinity, and they have three children.

# Because You Already Have the Scars

## Aleta Payne McClenney

In my dream, I am once again being wheeled toward emergency surgery, a sweet nurse assuring me that I'm going to be fine, the doctor explaining what will happen if the operation indeed reveals a pregnancy growing somewhere it shouldn't be. Fighting breathless panic, I break through the static of their voices.

"But you've already done this! I've already had this operation," I argue. "Why are you doing this again?"

The answer propels me awake: "Because you already have the scars."

It has been almost twenty years since I doubled over at work, sliced through by pain that gradually eased but left me gray and shaking. The next days were marked by a misdiagnosis, recurring pain, an ambulance.

"Do you have any children at home?" a doctor asked. I remember her as being the kind one, patiently and gently explaining that this pregnancy probably would not end with a baby, and without immediate surgery, the three-year-old and one-year-old boys at home might lose their mother.

I hadn't realized I was expecting. But within minutes, I learned that I was and that the pregnancy almost certainly could not continue. If, during surgery, they found a viable fetus unrelated to the source of my pain, I would wake up pregnant. If, as they suspected, it were growing outside of my uterus, they would save my life.

Perhaps if I'd had more time to think about it, I would have prayed. But in the precious moments as I faced the probability of saying everything I would ever say to the hope of a baby growing within me, I spoke only to that hope. The two older brothers at home. The dog who appreciated children as endless sources of dropped food.

The grandparents, the father, the mom who would give anything in that moment to offer a chance at life.

I woke up to an ungentle doctor who offered pictures of my insides, clinical explanations, and assurances that the procedure had gone well. Logically, I understood his words and was grateful for a healthy prognosis. Emotionally, "well" seemed profane.

The worst of the nightmares and anxiety persisted for months, until just about the time we would have welcomed a new baby. The physical scars have faded, and the sadness has dulled—still there, but without that sharp edge.

I was only aware of being pregnant for a handful of hours, most of those sedated. But those hours changed me. The physical scars have faded, but others remain. My life has been richly blessed by three sons, one of them born after the loss. My gratitude to God for them is profound, but there will forever be regret in my mother's heart for the hope I could not sustain.

## Prayer

God, who loves us infinitely as a parent loves a child, comfort us in our times of despair and loss, sustain us in our times of recovery and hope, and remind us that we learn both from joy and from grief. Amen.

**Aleta Payne McClenney** has worked as a writer and editor for newspapers and magazines. She is currently a freelance writer and non-profit professional. Aleta and her husband have three sons, ages 22, 20, and 16.

# Grief Out of Season

## Christopher Ingram

> *My soul is bereft of peace; I have forgotten what happiness is.... But this I call to mind, and therefore I have hope: The steadfast love of the* Lord *never ceases, his mercies never come to an end; they are new every morning; great is your faithfulness. "The* Lord *is my portion," says my soul, "therefore I will hope in him." The* Lord *is good to those who wait for him, to the soul that seeks him.* (Lamentations 3:17, 21-25, NRSV)

I have a friend whose first child was born with numerous special medical needs. We call him a "million-dollar baby," though his health care has certainly cost several millions of dollars. His early childhood has required dozens of surgeries, therapies, and trips to specialists around the country. I never once saw or heard his family complain about the sacrifices they made on a daily basis for his care.

When their second child was born years later, my friend told me how the birth of a healthy child cast his memory of their experience raising their first child in a whole new light. With nothing to compare to their first experience, they had always taken the next steps with their "million-dollar baby" naively unaware of just how hard their journey was. Paradoxically, the gift of a healthy sibling was a source of deep sadness for them: as they found simpler patterns of living with the new baby, they were able to grieve the reality of how different, and difficult, life had been for their family thus far.

In *A Whole New World: Life After Bethany*, Jan Rush recalls the tears she shed in her hospital room immediately after the birth of her son, Samuel. She cried tears of joy over welcoming a new life into her family. At the same time, those tears expressed deep grief for her daughter Bethany, born ten years before, who had been killed in a car accident. Conventional wisdom says, "Be happy, your child is here," but Rush's response rings true. In the midst of one of the best days of her life, "the wave of grief had come very unexpectedly, a reminder of the cyclical nature of grief."

I was lost when our family experienced miscarriage. I hardly believed that the pregnancy was even real. I didn't know how to listen or speak to my spouse. She, who had experienced it all so fully in her body, and I, from the outside looking in, could not make a meaningful connection with what had happened.

It was only years later, when we welcomed a newborn child into our family, that I more fully understood the loss for my wife—and for me. His arrival was an occasion for joy, to be sure, and also the first real occasion for me to mourn the loss of our first child years before. As the refrains of Louise Bogan's "Song for the Last Act" poignantly sing,

*Now that I have your face by heart, I look . . .*
*Now that I have your voice by heart, I read . . .*
*Now that I have your heart by heart, I see . . .*

Sometimes, God's good gifts bid grief to arrive out of season: a deferred dream comes to pass, a returning sense of balance or normalcy to living life, a restored relationship, a new hope or new opportunity comes your way. Sometimes, it is their goodness that reminds us of our sadness, and these gifts speak directly to our grief with the assurance of God's provision for today and beyond.

The deep pains of life can be healed and redeemed because the faithfulness of God shows up, not to erase or invalidate our pain but to remind us that God meets us where we are and grants us a future. Today's prayer from Lamentations shows how holding the gifts and pains of life together before God is a powerful act of trust that allows us to experience the faithfulness of God. Let that unfailing love bless you and keep you. Amen.

## Prayer

"My soul is bereft of peace; I have forgotten what happiness is. . . . But this I call to mind, and therefore I have hope: The steadfast love of the LORD never ceases, his mercies never come to an end; they are new every morning; great is your faithfulness. 'The LORD is my portion,' says my soul, 'therefore I will hope in him.' The LORD is good to those who wait for him, to the soul that seeks him. Amen." (Lam 3:17, 21-25)

> A native of Fredericksburg, Virginia, **Christopher Ingram** is married to Jeanell Cox, a CBF-endorsed health-care chaplain, and he is a father to three young sons. He is a graduate of the University of Virginia and Duke Divinity School. Over the course of his journey, he has served in ministries with the Virginia prison system, two congregations in Germany, and as an educator and pastor to congregations in Raleigh, Smithfield, and Elizabeth City, North Carolina. Currently, he serves as the senior pastor of Yates Baptist Church in Durham, North Carolina.

# My God, My God, Why . . . ?

## GAIL POWERY

In March 2011, we learned that we were expecting our third child. My previous pregnancies were normal, so I thought I knew what to expect. A little less than two weeks before I was scheduled to have my official doctor's visit, I started feeling different. I wasn't hurting or in any discomfort. I wasn't spotting or bleeding, but I felt strange. I didn't feel pregnant. I called my doctor, and she immediately scheduled an ultrasound for the next morning. After the ultrasound, the nurse took me into the doctor's office while my doctor was sitting at her desk. She looked up at me and shook her head. It was not good news.

The doctor explained that I was about eleven weeks pregnant with twins, but one of the twins had died. The other was fighting to stay alive. The heartbeat was very low. We hoped for a miracle and waited one more week to have another ultrasound to check the other baby, but the idea of waiting was devastating. I did everything I could to hold myself together, knowing that I was carrying death and life at the same time within me. I cried, and tears were my food as I questioned, "God, why?"

I told my husband, and he was shocked by it all—twins and one baby dead? My God, why? Who would have thought that we would have twins and then lose one? How could I continue for another week knowing that I was carrying life and death inside me? It was a long, emotional week for us. Our family and friends prayed for a miracle. I hung on to hope.

Then the day arrived for the second ultrasound. My husband and I hoped for good news. I had the ultrasound and went into the doctor's office. Again, I saw her face, and I knew that life had ended.

She confirmed that I had lost both of my babies. All she could do was say, "Sorry."

There was no visible reason why my babies died.

There was nothing the doctor could say to make sense of what had happened. And now, the only thing she could do was schedule to remove my two babies from my body. Sorrow and anger ricocheted in my heart. Why, God? Why? Why couldn't you save my babies? Like the Psalmist, like Jesus, I cried, "My God, my God, why have you forsaken me?" (Ps 22:1).

There are no easy answers to the question, "Why?" But like those who have gone before me, I can still say "my" God and remain in relationship with God, even when I'm angry or grieving. There are no questions too hard for God. This question of lament, like many of the lament psalms, is voiced in hope because it is asked in God's presence to a living God. God is there in the lament, in the question, and even when you are searching for answers. And, like the ending of Psalm 22, I can still say today, "I shall live for God."

This is not to say that it has not been a tough journey that will continue to bring strange grief at unexpected times. When that grief arrives, for you, for me, may this be our prayer:

## Prayer

God from whom I live, even when life has been taken from my very body, "my heart is sick" (Jer 8:18). I have asked "why," but no reason has made itself known. You see more than I can. You understand more than I know. Take my questions as expressions of faith from one who doesn't claim to have all the answers but knows Who does. Like a parent who consoles a hurting child, God, console me. Hear me when I cry, as Christ did on the cross. God, you are always there, even in my questions—"my God." I don't understand and may never know why, but you do because I pray, as Christ prayed on the cross, "My God, my God, why . . . ?" And you hear me and love me still. Amen.

**Gail Powery** lives in Durham, North Carolina, where she worships with her family at Duke University

Chapel. She has a Bachelor of Arts degree with a major in Psychology and a minor in Sociology from Southeastern University. She spent much of her career working with homeless youth ages 13–21 who were substance abusers. Currently, she spends most of her time volunteering at her children's school and serving on various committees there.

# The Mourning Is Never Far Off

Blake Hart

*Blessed are those who mourn, for they will be comforted.* (Matthew 5:4)

I keep thinking that at some point this will get easier, and to a certain extent it does. We settle into a new life. It's not the life we had before or the life we would have experienced were Silas here with us—it's just a new, different life.

The pain, though, is always there. It's never far off, and the most random of situations bring it to the fore. Cheering on my favorite teams during the World Cup, realizing that Silas should be here with me, wearing a matching jersey and repeating the chants after me. Splashing in a kiddie pool on the Fourth of July, noticing the absence of his small but joyful laughter. For that matter, celebrating any holiday, realizing that our celebrations will always be one person short.

When the pain comes, so do the tears, and I always hope that one day they won't arrive. That I won't have to feel ashamed of my tears, of my grief, or of my mourning. Men shouldn't cry, I have been known to tell myself, especially while they're in the grocery store looking at flowers for their son's grave. I'm reminded of Jesus' words: "Blessed are those who mourn . . . ."

That seems confusing, though, because those of us who mourn don't really feel blessed. But I guess it doesn't have much to do with how I feel. It has much more to do with the fact that Jesus declares a blessing over us in the midst of our mourning.

Jesus blesses us when we realize that the realities of this world are not as God originally intended. Jesus blesses us when we realize that wars aren't part of the plan, that death and destruction are distant from God's desires, that cancer, AIDS, and heart failure are intruders on God's good Earth. Jesus blesses not only because we realize this but also because we mourn. We feel the pain and the heartache of a world gone awry.

At times, that mourning cuts too close to home. Even then, Jesus blesses us because we realize that children aren't supposed to die before their parents. Mothers and fathers aren't supposed to come home from the hospital with empty arms and even emptier hearts.

I wonder why Jesus says this. Why does he declare us blessed while we're in the depths of grief? Shouldn't it be that Jesus blesses us by turning our mourning into dancing? The only thing I can figure is that mourning comes from love. The depths of our heartache and despair serve to expose the depths of our love and affection. We mourn greatly because we love greatly.

I guess that true pain would be the absence of any emotion. If I felt nothing at the thought of Silas and the empty places left by his death, that would be agony. Instead, I mourn, I grieve, and I cry because I love, and, knowing that love is never-ending, I hope for the day when my love is expressed not through tears of sadness but through an embrace of love.

Receive, then, this blessing from Jesus: "Blessed are those who mourn, for they will be comforted."

## Prayer

God of love, our mourning serves as a sign of our love, and since you are a God of love, including a love for us, it must mean that you mourn greatly with us as well. Help us to find solace in that truth. Amen.

**Blake Hart** and his wife, Bekah, lost their firstborn son, Silas Jeremey, on November 7, 2013, while living in Chile. They now live in South Carolina with their second son, Benjamin. Blake serves as the Missions Coordinator for the Cooperative Baptist Fellowship of South Carolina.

# Grieving for and with Our Child

## Rebekah McLeod Hutto and William Joseph (B. J.) Hutto

When Rebekah's water broke at twenty weeks and our baby girl, Mary, died on December 9, we were devastated. It was a grief beyond metaphors. Not only did we mourn her absence; we also had to reckon with her presence. We had to pack up and remove the pictures, videos, and reminders we'd already collected during those five months of pregnancy. Foremost among these was the video recording of us telling our three-year-old daughter, Hannah Ruth, that she would soon be a big sister. Hannah Ruth was overcome with excitement; she overflowed with questions: "Can I hold her?" "Can I name her?" "When will she be here?" "Can I teach her to dance?"

Thus, when we returned home from the hospital that December weekend, another devastating reality was waiting for us: we had to tell Hannah Ruth that she wouldn't be a big sister. This was heartbreaking. Grieving ourselves, we listened to her grief and tried to answer her questions. You see, we wanted another baby largely because of Hannah Ruth. While we, as parents, wanted to grow our family, we also wanted to offer the gift of a sibling to our first daughter. This spunky, determined extrovert wasn't created to be an only child. She clings to her friends and her friends' siblings. She constantly plays with babies in the nursery. Telling her that her baby sister had died was one of the hardest things either of us has ever had to do.

The conversation we had with Hannah Ruth that afternoon became a running conversation over the next weeks and months. She told everyone she knew—and some whom she'd just met—that we had a baby that died. She asked more questions: "Will I ever be a big sister?" "Where did our baby go?" "When will we have a baby that doesn't die?" We were asking ourselves these questions, too, but she was relentless, desperately trying to make sense of what happened. Temper tantrums followed the questions. Realizing our sadness and doubt along with her own, sometimes all she could do was lash out in anger.

And why should she not? As a therapist told us, "She's having the temper tantrums you two wish you could have." But there were also other times when Hannah Ruth would hug us and say, "We'll have another baby someday." She began climbing into bed and gently stroking Rebekah's cheek, telling her that she loved her and that it would all be all right. Sadness, confusion, anger, empathy—this is how our little girl grieved. None of this was easy for us, but watching Hannah Ruth grieve was particularly painful for our already weary hearts.

However, we've also come to realize that Hannah Ruth is teaching us something about grief. Just when we think we've turned a page, she turns up with another question, another matter-of-fact statement about grief, about how reality has changed for her with the death of her baby sister. You don't get over a death like this, and Hannah Ruth forces us to admit that. As the developmental experts have told us, she will re-grieve this loss as she gets older. But won't we all? Sometimes you just need to ask all the questions that people tell you are not helpful. Sometimes you need to lash out in anger and scream at what has happened. Sometimes you need to be matter-of-fact with how you're feeling, what you're going through, how life will never be the same. Some wounds, doctors tell us, heal best with sunlight; they have to be exposed.

We, too, re-grieve what has happened. It has changed us as individuals, our relationships with one another, and our understanding of our life together. Sometimes, just when we think we're doing better, the grief will rise to the surface and spill over in tears. Things set us off: Advent, baby clothes, infants who would have been—should have been—Mary's age, the young, lonely sisters in *Frozen*. Every time we see Hannah Ruth playing with someone else's baby or someone else's sibling, every time we hear the word "sisters," we're reminded of what was lost in our daughter's death.

But some things remain. The grief never goes away. It remains. We remain, too, as does God. And Hannah Ruth, more than anyone else, reminds us of all of these things.

## Prayer

Life-giving God,
We grieve the death of hopes we anticipated, dreams we envisioned, and a relationship we desired.
Where there was sweet expectation, now there is bitter disappointment.
Allow us, O God, to grieve and accept this loss.
Warm us with the embrace of your arms;
knit together our frayed emotions, and bind our hearts with the fabric of your love.
Fill us with hope in the good and loving name of Jesus, Amen.

Note: The book *Talking with Children about Loss* by Maria Trozzi is an excellent developmental guide on children and grief. It's a secular resource but one we've found incredibly helpful in our own family and with others.

**Rebekah Hutto** is the Associate Minister of Christian Education and Discipleship at Brick Presbyterian Church in New York City. Originally from Greenville, South Carolina, Rebekah is serving her second call in ordained ministry at Brick. She is married to **B. J. Hutto**, an ordained Baptist pastor, originally from Orangeburg, South Carolina. Having served two churches, B. J. is currently completing his PhD in theological ethics (at-distance) at King's College, Aberdeen. They live in New York City with their daughter, Hannah Ruth.

# Throwing My Anger at God

## Jenny Barrier

*Therefore I will not restrain my mouth;*
*I will speak in the anguish of my spirit;*
*I will complain in the bitterness of my soul.* (Job 7:11)

"God, I am mad. No, I am furious, irate. And you know what, God? I am mad at you. I have so much anger inside me right now, God, that I don't know what to do with it. So, God, I'm going to be angry at you because you're the only one I know large enough to handle this much pain and this much fury."

This is a rough transcript of a prayer I once prayed. The original was probably longer, and I know it included some choice swear words. My prayer was far from being as eloquent as Job's complaint to God, but both prayers came from a place of deep pain. I prayed this prayer about two weeks after I found out that my husband and I had lost our first baby. I had happily gone to my obstetrician's office for my twelve-week appointment. I was excited to have my first ultrasound and finally see my child. Instead, I found out that my baby had stopped developing weeks before, but my body had not realized this. My stomach had begun to grow. I was nauseated and exhausted. I had all the signs of a healthy pregnancy except the most important: a growing baby.

In the following days and weeks I felt a barrage of emotions: grief, loss of hope, helplessness. What I felt most of all, however, was an overwhelming sense of betrayal. My body had betrayed me, fooling me into singing at night to a child who was not there, into rubbing my belly when I thought no one was looking. The bigger betrayal, though, came from God. Bible verses like Jeremiah 29:11 that once held promise now seemed to be full of cruel mockery: "For surely I know the plans I have for you, says the LORD, plans for your welfare and not for harm, to give you a future with hope." I felt harmed. My hope seemed to have evaporated.

My feelings of betrayal filled me with anger. This was a burning, almost soul-crushing anger. My body did not feel strong enough to contain such rage. So, as I prayed my prayer, I did not hold back. Like Job, I complained in the bitterness of my soul. I balled up all the anger I felt inside of me, all my feelings of betrayal, and I threw them at God. Part of me wanted to hurt God just as much as I was hurting. The rest of me just wanted to find a safe place to put the rage, somewhere that it could not harm me or my husband.

I would like to say that this prayer healed me. It didn't. I still felt betrayed, and I was still mad. Even as I write this seven years later, I find myself crying as I relive the experience. The grief can still be raw. It would have been foolish to expect instant comfort; it took Job forty-two chapters to reach a new equilibrium. What my prayer did, however, was start the long process of healing. I began to feel like I could breathe again. Eventually I was able to pray again, too.

Recently, my Sunday school class was discussing the topic of prayer and one theologian's statement that all prayer is based in gratitude. One person asked if there could be gratitude in lament. I told an abbreviated account of my conversation with God, and as I was talking I had a realization: even my lament to God, my anger at God, had an element of gratitude at its core. I had no gratitude that I lost my baby. I am not, nor will I ever be, grateful for that. Instead, even as I was in the depths of my anger, I knew where to turn. God took my rage and, instead of judging me for it, absorbed it into God's self. I will be forever grateful that God was big enough to take and hold my anger when it was too big for me.

## *Prayer*

Gracious God, thank you that you are with us even in the midst of our anger and hurt. Hold us, sustain us, support us. Amen.

**Jenny Barrier** is a member of Watts Street Baptist Church in Durham, North Carolina. There, she has been a part of the Hannah Ministry, where dreaming about Project Pomegranate first began. She is a graduate of the Baptist Theological Seminary at Richmond and is also a specialist in Russian studies. She spends her time mothering two boys, volunteering at church, and knitting.

# And then the Anger Came . . .

## Joanne Henley

And then the anger came, from nowhere and everywhere all at the same time. I had no name for it, nor any real direction that I wanted to send it. Was I angry at God? Was I angry at myself? Was I angry at this baby who left me without a real vision of her or his presence? Why was I so mad? The anger, my anger, did not make sense to me.

It had been months since my first two miscarriages. They were early, in that time between the joy of discovering new life and the awe of hearing the heartbeat of it. Somehow, because I lost my babies so early, I felt like it should hurt less. Less than what, I don't know. I had friends and family who had lost babies much later in their pregnancies. I had, at that point in my career, witnessed countless parents saying good-bye to their children in the emergency room and the pediatric and neonatal intensive care units. So perhaps the heartwrenching grief of those parents was my comparison. All of those people lost "more" than I did. My babies weren't even babies yet. No one had called me mom. No one had recognized me as a mother. Those two little lives obviously didn't have what they needed to grow, and so they didn't. I hadn't actually lost that much. Why was I so mad?

Comparison is rarely helpful in grief. What is helpful are freedom and grace, the unconditional acceptance of every feeling, even anger, as it comes. The pain of losing my baby before he or she was a baby, of never being called mom and of wondering whether I would ever be known as a mother was exactly why it hurt so bad. The anger that came let out the anguish, disappointment, guilt, confusion, love, and doubt I felt in those months, like the air leaving a balloon with a pinprick.

Today, my memory of that anger still ties me to the intensity of my grief. I did not know then what I know now. I did not know that before the next year ended, I would give birth to a precious little girl. I did not know that there would be one more miscarriage after her birth and then no more pregnancies. What I did know was that the grief of miscarriage was unlike any other grief I had experienced. Six years later, that is still the case.

Along the way, I have found the closing verses from a prayer by Ted Loder in *Guerrillas of Grace* particularly helpful.[1] They have tethered me to solid ground when I thought my grief and anger might just carry me away. May this be your prayer today.

## Prayer

Eternal One,
. . . Enfold me now in your presence;
Restore to me your peace;
Renew me through your power;
And ground me in your grace.
Amen.

### Note

1. Ted Loder, *Guerrillas of Grace: Prayers for the Battle* (Minneapolis: Augsburg Books, 1981) 11.

**Joanne Henley** is a board-certified chaplain working at Novant Health Derrick L. Davis Cancer Center. She is a graduate of the Divinity School at Wake Forest University. Joanne is married to Tommy, and they enjoy the precious gift of raising their daughter, Ashleigh.

# Beyond the Silence

## Chris Barrett

> *. . . the Spirit helps us in our weakness; for we do not know how to pray as we ought, but that very Spirit intercedes with sighs too deep for words.* (Romans 8:26)

Augustine once described us preachers as peddlers of words. I was a novice word-peddler when we had our first miscarriage. And in those moments of pain, I ran slam out of my own words. That is not to say that no words came to me. But they weren't my words. Nor were they words that I actually spoke aloud.

The words that came to me most frequently in that dim season were these: "the Spirit helps us in our weakness; for we do not know how to pray as we ought, but that very Spirit intercedes with sighs too deep for words." It was these words of Paul that gave me permission to take leave of words for a while, to lean into the dark mysteries of loss, pain, and grief without words getting in the way.

It didn't matter that this sentence was originally penned by Paul, a bachelor itinerant preacher who almost certainly never struggled with the loss my wife and I were experiencing. What did matter was that these words, more than any other, gave me consolation. They consoled me because they lifted the burden I felt to interpret the loss in real time and in my own words—first to myself, then to my family, and finally to my churches. They comforted me because they promised that even as I failed to find words that would carry the freight of my raw emotions, God received my inchoate moans as prayers. I found deep reassurance from Paul's promise that even when I didn't understand what was happening around me or within me, even when bitter tears flowed more readily than words, God's own Spirit was faithfully conveying my heart's needs and desires to God's heart.

Part of my difficulty with finding words was due to feeling helpless. I watched as Elise endured the physical as well as the emotional anguish of the miscarriage. It was her abdomen and legs that were wracked with cramps, and it was her body that endured invasive tests and painful procedures. It was she who felt the reality of the miscarriage as a corporeal loss. I stood by, gripped with my own grief, horrified at the all-encompassing nature of Elise's pain.

In the face of her profound physical, spiritual, and emotional suffering, I felt as if my role was to speak as little as possible and be present as fully as possible. Looking back, I believe that I also felt some guilt. It was our relating as husband and wife that had led to this pain, and now Elise bore the greater part. This is fine and good when there's a new creation at the end of the suffering. But when there is an empty womb and an empty crib, the pain seems all the more harshly uneven. And since I'd had cancer and radiation treatment in the past, my head was full of questions about whether something about my contribution had led to this happening.

Flooded by these internal uncertainties, I found myself wanting to hug Elise. A lot. I would have said then that I was offering those hugs to console her. And that was true, as far as it went. I understand now that in addition to seeking to help Elise by hugging her, I needed her hugs as much or more than she needed mine.

I would encourage all partners of a woman who has experienced a miscarriage to examine the care you offer. Make sure you're crystal clear about how much is for your partner and how much is about trying to meet your own need for comfort. There will always be some of both. That is the nature of a mutually supportive marriage. But now, years later, I see that precisely because of the unevenness of the experience between spouses, a supportive partner's job is to keep the ledger balanced in favor of what feels kind and comforting to the person who endures the lion's share of the suffering.

Which brings me back to words. My muteness in the face of our loss was an important anchor for me. I believe it was precisely the right way to respond to the miscarriage, especially early on. It helped me lean on God and interact with Elise instinctively and compassionately in the deepest darkness of our shared grief.

Here's the thing. In the eleven years since our first miscarriage, these words are the first I've ever written on the subject. Sure, I've thought about it. I've talked about it, though infrequently. I even helped edit my wife's book about it. But until now, I don't think I've processed my own feelings sufficiently to move beyond the silence. The toll that has taken on me and my marriage is a story that's still being written. Falling silent can see you through the funnel of a tornado, but cleaning up the debris, rebuilding in the storm's wake, will almost always require patience, discipline, and, yes, words.

## *Prayer*

God of Sacred Silence, bring comfort to the souls, hearts, bodies, and minds of those who have suffered loss. When our words fail, give us the surpassing comfort of your Word Drawn Near. Make your grace real to those in the midst of pain, and bring us to your peace. As you came in the fullness of time to deliver us through Jesus Christ, meet us again in our places of emptiness. Restore us to the hope to which we were called, hope born of the suffering through which you have promised always to accompany us. Amen.

> **Chris Barrett** is pastor at St. James United Methodist Church in Spartanburg, South Carolina. He and his wife, Elise, also a United Methodist pastor, suffered a series of pregnancy losses over several years, which led to her writing the book *What Was Lost: A Christian Journey through Miscarriage*. In 2013, Chris underwent a bone marrow transplant for the treatment of non-Hodgkin's lymphoma. He chronicled his journey at http://marrowchristianity.blogspot.com/.

# When They Want Me to Speak

## Rick Jordan

I had been visiting the young couple for several days. Their infant was in the neonatal intensive care unit, not doing well. I was the chaplain over this unit. After a few days, they heard the doctor say to them what they most feared and didn't want to hear: "We did everything we could, but your baby didn't make it."

I was called to the unit. The couple was rocking their baby, saying their good-byes. I sat with them in silence. *When they want me to speak, they'll ask me*, I thought. And they did, engaging me in their very different forms of grief.

"Isn't he beautiful?" the mother asked.

"Yes, beautiful," I responded.

After a while, she said, "Will we ever know why?"

"Would that help?" I asked.

She paused. "Maybe . . . I guess not. It's going to hurt no matter what." Then she said to her child, "I'm going to love you and miss you no matter what."

The father was quiet during our time together. He was loving and supportive. He held the baby. He stroked his wife's back. He wiped tears from his cheek. But he remained quiet.

Sometimes, that's the way it is: the partner's role is simply to be present and supportive. His grief is expressed in the love he demonstrates to the sorrowful mother. The months of pregnancy were different for him. He was not confronted with morning sickness or kicks within or comments from strangers about a changing body—things that she had experienced as constant reminders of a new life on the way. He dealt with her illness and felt some of the kicks and noticed her body's redevelopment, but it was not the daily, sudden, surprising experience it was for her. Both had dreams for their new child. Both talked about names. Both wondered aloud about the color and curl and length of hair. But the last few months were different for each of them. The grieving will be different as well.

When she stepped out for a few minutes, he began articulating to me his struggle.

"I feel bad that I don't feel as bad as her."

"You think you should have as much sadness as she does?" I asked.

"Shouldn't I?" he said. "I mean, this is my child, too. . . . I wish things were different. I wish I could just make him live and we could walk out of this place happy, like we were supposed to."

"That was your expectation, your dream, but now it's gone."

"Yes . . . but we're going to make it through this."

"You want to move on past this."

"It won't help to linger. I mean, I hate this happened, and it is sad, but you've got to play the hand you're dealt."

"The way you want to play this hand and the way she needs to play this hand may be different."

"That's true. That's true."

The mother entered the room again and took the baby from her husband's arms. We sat in silence. She wept quietly. He had one hand on the baby and one on her hand. Then, he asked me to speak. For them. To God.

## Prayer

Creator God, when our creations do not turn out the way we planned, we feel shock and anger and sadness. This is so hard when our creation was a child. Help us to be sensitive to another's expression of loss. Help us to know that there is no standard way to experience or express our grief, so that we neither elevate nor discount another's processing of pain. Amen.

**Rick Jordan** is the Church Resources Coordinator for the Cooperative Baptist Fellowship of North Carolina. As a chaplain resident at Spartanburg (South Carolina) General Hospital, Rick started a SHARE support group for grieving parents. A few years later as Associate Pastor at Viewmont Baptist Church in Hickory, North Carolina, Rick and a United Methodist pastor began The Pregnancy Loss Support Group. He shares this story about an experience that has shaped his own ministry.

# It's Not Okay

## Ryan R. Whitley

> *O Lord, God of my salvation, when, at night, I cry out in your presence, let my prayer come before you; incline your ear to my cry. For my soul is full of troubles, and my life draws near to Sheol. I am counted among those who go down to the Pit; I am like those who have no help.* (Psalm 88:1-4)

I have come to this place, to this hospital room in the middle of this crisis, because I was called in. Because your loss is a significant one. I have been praying for you even though I have not met you before now. As a priest, I am often called to this place when things do not go as planned, when things take a turn so far away from what was hoped. Even though I have been here many times before, I have never heard your grief. I have never cried with you. I want you to know that I consider this meeting sacred, because you are sacred to God and because your child is sacred to God. This grief is sacred, though unwelcome.

There is no grief like your grief. No sorrow like your sorrow. And I cannot fix that. I cannot make that go away. What I can do is sit with you in your sackcloth and ashes. I promise you that. I promise you that I can be present with you in the midst of the awful, horrible grief that is in this room, and we need not be polite about how awful and horrible it really is.

What's happened to you isn't right or fair. And it is not something that you need to carry yourself, or from which you need to protect me, or anyone else around you. The truth of the matter is, we, God's priests, have walked through the valley of the shadow of death before. We know how scary it is. And so it is okay for you to say that you're scared, or sad, or pissed off. It's okay to say that this is not okay. Go ahead, you won't offend me, and you certainly won't offend God.

God, who made the heavens and the earth and everything that is in them, can take your anger. Do you need to cry? Go ahead. Do you need to yell? Go ahead. Do you need to be silent? Go ahead. I can sit with you in all of that. I can walk with you through this particular valley of the shadow of death. I am here to remind you of the promise that God is with you, closer to you now than perhaps ever before. You are beautiful in God's sight. Your baby is beautiful in God's sight. You are loved. And you are never alone.

You know that this is not as it should be. And you're right. It is not okay. But you will survive. And I will sit with you until you feel like you can breathe again. And when I leave, I will not forget you. Because God will not forget you. God knows it's okay not to be okay.

## Prayer

Oh my God, help me. Help me when I feel like I cannot breathe. Help me when I feel like I cannot speak. Help me know that you are with me, that your Spirit is in this place, and that when I cry, you cry with me. Give me the courage I will need to face the days and times to come, and the companions who will walk with me. Grant me the grace to accept their help. Please be near to me, O God, and let me feel your presence, for you are my help and my salvation. Amen.

**Ryan R. Whitley** is an Episcopal priest serving as the Rector of The Nevil Memorial Church of St. George, in Ardmore, Pennsylvania, just outside of Philadelphia. In addition to his parish and diocesan duties, Fr. Ryan spends a lot of time at the hospital. He has served for the past several years on the Schwartz Rounds committee at Lankenau Hospital (which provides an avenue for health care providers to discuss the emotional impact of critical cases) and has also served there on the planning committee for the Grandin Lectures, a lecture series seeking to explore the intersection of faith and health care. However, his most rewarding time at Lankenau is that spent as a volunteer emergency chaplain in the labor and delivery department. Fr. Ryan is married with one son, and a daughter on the way.

# Weary with My Moaning

## Sheree Jones

> *I am weary with my moaning; every night I flood my bed with tears; I drench my couch with my weeping. My eyes waste away because of the grief. . . .* (Psalm 6:6-7a)

I have seen this wasting grief of Psalm 6. I have steeled myself against the moaning, wading through the floods of tears. As a hospital chaplain, I am called to provide support and comfort to the family who has experienced the death of a child. And each time I am called to be with such a family, I find myself struggling to bring comfort to those who have experienced such great loss. Just this week, I have been called to the bedside of three such families, and the depth of emotion and pain was evident on the faces of everyone present.

Each time that I enter into this grief, I am struck by how often we humans try to be strong for others. We may attempt to hide, or deny, our true feelings not only from others (and even ourselves) but also from the One who knows us best, the One who created us and instilled in us the ability to feel great joy and great sadness. In the midst of such great pain, it is difficult to be honest about what we are feeling and experiencing, and it is difficult to give ourselves permission to feel it.

When a loss like this occurs, the depth of the emotions, the intensity of the grief, cannot fully be expressed with words. The clearest expression of our pain can only come through the shedding of tears. It is as the psalmist says: with moaning, tears, and weeping, we come to God. These words from the psalmist give us hope that our God wants to hear our feelings and receive our tears; that God is about more than simply taking our tears away; that God will be with us as we cry, as we moan with the grief that has no words.

God wants us to be real. God does not want us to hold back. God wants us to be honest with our struggles and our sorrows. It is in our authenticity that we experience the true nature of our Creator, the compassion and presence of one who knows us so intimately. We experience the closeness and the comfort that our Creator wants to give us.

In Psalm 6:9, the psalmist goes on to say "The LORD has heard my supplication," and those words empower us with the knowledge that no matter the heartache, the grief, the loss, our God hears us and is present with us in the midst of it. When words fail to express our grief, God hears what we wish we could say. And God sits with us in our pain and walks with us on the journey.

## Prayer

Ever-present God, hear the cries of those who grieve. Give them courage to feel their pain, to speak their truth and be comforted by you. As they move forward, assure them of your presence in the midst of their sorrow. Amen.

**Sheree Jones** serves as a staff chaplain with Novant Health Forsyth Medical Center in Winston-Salem, North Carolina.

# Not Ready to Face the World

## Joy M. Freeman

> *But they that wait upon the* LORD *shall renew their strength; they shall mount up with wings as eagles, they shall run and not be weary, and they shall walk and not faint.* (Isaiah 40:31)

"God I'm not ready. I do not want to see a baby yet. It hurts too much. I do not want to say congratulations to the new parents I'm about to see." These thoughts stayed with me as I prepared to go back to work as a hospital chaplain just a week after we said good-bye to our baby, Hope.

I had barely started to put my world back together. I was not ready to deal with the deep jealousy that came whenever I saw a mother with a baby. So I was less than prepared when another mother, who was dropping her child off at daycare at the same time I dropped off my oldest daughter, asked me to hold her baby as she helped her older child with something. I wanted to say "no," yet I was too emotionally weak to deal with the fall-out or conversation that might come with me saying no. So I grudgingly said "sure" as I reached out to hold that little baby. I did not need to hold the little one for long, but it was the start to facing my jealousy. I waited another week before going back to serve as the chaplain on the maternity unit, in hopes that I would be better off.

But grief hardly ever agrees to go along with our timeline, or so I found out as I faced those ugly, dark feelings of jealousy. How in the world could I, as a chaplain, a representative of God and that which is spiritual, do my work on the maternity unit, being happy for these new parents, giving comfort to scared parents when all I wanted to do was scream "At least you have a baby"?

At this time, I remembered a verse that I have clung to in other times of distress and difficulty. Isaiah 40:31 has long been a favorite of mine, and again it served as a reminder that if I did not try to get through those hours on the maternity unit alone, but instead asked God to go with me, I just might make it through the day. It did not change the way I felt, but at least that reminder made it possible for me to do my work without completely falling apart.

Time is important. The time I spent waiting for the deep ache of missing baby Hope to subside was not wasted time. The time I spent waiting for the jealousy toward new parents to lessen was not wasted time. My grief would not be so raw forever. I needed time to honor those deep feelings. I needed time to begin to let go of the darkness and find my own place of strength again, so that I could get back to marveling at and celebrating the miracle of new life and birth; so that I could begin, again, to extend God's grace—grace that I had experienced myself—to those who would need it themselves.

First, I had to be willing to walk through my grief, trusting that God was walking with me, keeping me from fainting under the sheer weight of it. For me, it all started with doing what I did not want to do, but for some reason knew I had to do: hold a newborn baby.

We each have our own moment of saying, "God, I'm not ready." As individuals, each moment is unique to our own situations. However, God's strength is waiting to help us walk and eventually get back to running our life-journey. It all starts with being able to say, "God, I'm not ready." God will carry us from there.

## *Prayer*

God of Grace, walk with these parents who are grieving, who may not even be able to see the day where they can look at a baby without crying deep tears of grief. Help them to know that you do not desire for them to hurt like this, that you cry with them. Surround them with your arms to give them the strength they need to begin to find the healing and wholeness you desire for them as they face their "I'm not ready" moment. Amen.

**Joy M. Freeman** graduated from Central Baptist Theological Seminary in 2001 with her Master of Divinity. She is an Endorsed American Baptist Chaplain and board-certified through the Association of Professional Chaplains. She serves as a Critical Care and Maternity Chaplain at North Kansas City Hospital in the Kansas City Metro Area. She is also a Veriditas Certified Labyrinth Facilitator.

# What a Friend . . .

## Erin K. McClain

> *What a friend we have in Jesus,*
> *All our sins and griefs to bear!*
> *What a privilege to carry*
> *Everything to God in prayer!* (Joseph M. Scriven, 1855)

> *"If this is how you treat your friends, it's no wonder you have so few of them."* (St. Teresa of Avila to God, after being thrown from her horse and landing in the mud)

October 15 always takes me by surprise. As a recurrent miscarrier—seven pregnancies but only one live birth—I'm prepped for Mother's Day and all the feelings it can evoke. I'm used to putting on a brave face for pregnancy announcements and baby showers. But October 15—Pregnancy and Infant Loss Remembrance Day, when you are supposed to light a candle at 7 p.m. to help create a wave of light around the world—gets me every year.

I've never been a good public griever. Though I bawl like a baby at weddings, I don't usually cry at funerals. As I learned not to calculate due dates until I was past the first trimester and grew more numb with each miscarriage, I sought to wrap my tattered dignity around myself and appear to be unaffected by the losses. As I threw myself into becoming pregnant again, surviving a rough pregnancy, parenting my daughter, and, ultimately, adopting my son, I stuffed my grief, anger, and disconnection from God further and further down until the shame and secret nature of the loss became internalized. Acknowledging or memorializing my body's failures seemed like a waste of time.

It was that same traitorous body that finally made me stop trying to hide my grief and anger from myself and God. After reluctantly participating in a service meant to honor the losses of infertility, where I felt my usual emotional and spiritual numbness when poking at the sore tooth of my pregnancy history, my rheumatoid arthritis flared and I ended up in bed for the next two days. As I lay there, I thought of St. Teresa lying in the mud and started to laugh/cry. "God, I'm starting to understand how she felt."

St. Teresa—whose feast day is, fittingly, October 15—wrote, "For prayer is nothing else than being on the terms of friendship with God." With my immobility, I had no way to busy away the realization that God and I had not been on friendly terms for a while. I was so mad that I didn't feel like I could pray. So I didn't. I just talked. Like God was a good girlfriend, I told God how disappointed and angry I was, how hard the losses had been, how I felt like my body was a failure. While I would love to say that the heavens opened and peace flowed over me like a river, the truth is that the conversation was stilted and I was still upset, though I did feel some small measure of peace.

God and I are still rebuilding our friendship. It becomes easier to talk to God each time I do it, and I am starting to own my story and my losses. The thought of openly acknowledging my grief seems less scary and more healing. The next time October 15 comes around, I'll have my candle ready.

## Prayer

Dear God, help us to remember that, like a good friend, you are always there to listen, even when we are not eloquent. Remind us that while you rejoice in our happiness, you are also strong enough to bear witness to our grief, anger, and shame. Help us to recall that all we have to do is start talking. Amen.

> **Erin K. McClain** is a bio-mama, an adoptive mama, and a maternal and child health program manager who lives in Durham, North Carolina. She has master's degrees in international affairs and public health, and she has experience working in civil society development, conflict resolution, and refugee resettlement in the United States and abroad, as well as promoting

the health of women and infants in the Southeast US. Erin is a member of Westminster Presbyterian Church in Durham, where she corrupts the youth (aka teaches Sunday school) and co-directs the Christmas pageant. She is also a member of the Project Pomegranate leadership team. She is an avid reader, baker, and music lover whose typical solution to a crappy day is a living room dance party followed by reading a favorite book while eating a high-calorie food.

# An Unlikely Prayer Partner

## Jennifer Andrews-Weckerly

*Here am I, the servant of the Lord; let it be with me according to your word.* (Luke 1:38)

"Have you considered praying with Mary?"

This was the question from my spiritual director when I finally broke down and told her what was *really* going on with me. I confessed that our inability to get pregnant had not brought me closer to God, but had in fact made me feel as though God were absent. Whenever I thought about lifting the burden to God, I had no words—mostly because I no longer trusted God.

But how could I turn to Mary? Mary didn't have to have sex to get pregnant or urinate on an ovulation stick to see if she carried a baby. What could she possibly have to offer me, and how could I possibly pray with a woman known worldwide for what happened in her womb? I left the session with my spiritual director incredulous, and half-wondering if she were not totally clueless.

Days later, with the proposal still lingering in my mind, I decided to look back at Scripture to see what it actually says about Mary. As I read, my anger softened. In Luke's Gospel, when Mary is told what will happen to her, she says, "Here am I, the servant of the Lord; let it be with me according to your word." Later, when shepherds come to visit, Luke says, "Mary treasured all these words and pondered them in her heart" (Luke 2:19). The more I read about Mary, the more I realized that although she is known most for whom she birthed, she never wanted to be pregnant or have a child—at least not at that time in her life. Her pregnancy happened *to* her, much like my inability to get pregnant was happening *to* me. Somehow she managed to trust that God would take care of her, even if she did not fully understand what was happening, and needed much time over the course of her life to ponder things in her heart.

So I began to pray with Mary. I held her hand as I prayed that I could be as trusting as she once was. I looked to her when I needed a feminine presence in my spiritual world, someone whom I knew might understand my pain. I went to Mary, hoping that someday I could also utter that promise: "Let it be with me according to your word." When I prayed with Mary, I did not see the victorious singer of the Magnificat (Luke 1:46-55); instead, I saw an uncertain woman on a scary journey with God.

Later that year, we became pregnant with our first child. We found out about the pregnancy right at the beginning of Advent—Mary's primary season! I remember as I held the news in secret, praying that nothing fatal would happen in that first trimester, how grateful I was to have Mary along this journey with me. I was slow to let God back in immediately. Mary was a great intercessor in those days. But I stood quietly with Mary that Advent, pondering the journey in my heart, praying with her that the pregnancy journey would be less fraught with anxiety than the attempting to get pregnant journey had been. I am forever changed by that prayer time with Mary, and I have turned to her in the years since that time. But mostly I am grateful to the wise spiritual director who was willing to risk alienating me with her challenge to pray in a new way.

## *Prayer*

Abiding God, though our hearts may know you are always with us, loving us, and caring for us, there are times when you feel treacherously absent. In those moments of abandonment, show us the light of your countenance, and rain your love down upon us. Help us to connect to those who have gone before us in the faith. In the name of your son, Jesus, we pray. Amen.

**Jennifer Andrews-Weckerly** joined the Episcopal Church of St. Margaret in December 2011 as the third rector in its forty-nine-year history. Prior to joining

St. Margaret's, she completed a Bachelor of Arts in Political Science at Duke University in 1999. After a year of AmeriCorps service in North Carolina, Jennifer served as the Director of Volunteer Services at Habitat for Humanity of New Castle County, Delaware, for almost six years. Jennifer earned her Master in Divinity from Virginia Theological Seminary in May 2009. Upon graduation, she served as the Curate and Assistant Rector at Christ Church Christiana Hundred in Delaware for more than two years. Jennifer is married and has two daughters. She enjoys spending time with her family and friends, traveling, watching movies, and squeezing in a yoga or zumba class when she can. Her blog can be found at http://seekingandserving.wordpress.com.

# Absence

## Stephanie McLeskey

*What is crooked cannot be made straight, and what is lacking cannot be counted.* (Ecclesiastes 1:15)

"I just know that it's all been worth it, now that you can look down into your daughter's beautiful face."

No.

It hasn't.

My daughter *is* beautiful. Motherhood is both wonderful and extremely hard. She is the result of my fifth pregnancy, and she is my first child. The losses have absolutely nothing to do with her, but all is not forgotten now that she is here. Three of the losses I grieve in the abstract—hopes dashed, dreams deferred. They were too early in the pregnancy for me to know their gender, for me to see a kicking foot, a beating heart. The other has a name.

I have not spoken his name aloud. It is not recorded on paper anywhere. In the moments after labor had ended, and paperwork was being filled out, and I was asked, "Do you have a name for him?" my voice caught. I glanced at my husband—we had not made that decision yet, so I only knew the name I was favoring at the time. I said no.

I also turned away from his tiny body, not able to bear seeing or holding the stillness that just hours before had been so active on the ultrasound screen. My body failed; his did not. He was healthy and perfect, but he was too small, too undeveloped, and so my faulty body ended his life before it had really begun.

I have been told the same thing I would tell anyone else: there is no fault. There is no need for guilt. There is nothing that could have been done differently, nothing that was known ahead of time that could have fixed this. My mind knows that. My heart still struggles.

And where was God? Again, my faith tells me that I was not targeted by an angry or vengeful God. My faith tells me that God did not cause these losses. In the dark, though, faith falters. It becomes a discipline. I asked myself the question, over and over—a mantra, a prayer, a lifeline: Where is God?

This I know: God was in the delivery room that day.

Even in the pain of the experience, I could feel the holiness of God's presence, the sacredness and awfulness of it. It was the compassion of Christ that flowed through the hands and the voice of my doctor, and the strength of Christ that sustained me through my husband's eyes locked with my own as I labored. Although we were still fairly new in town and very new to our church, it was by the grace of God that one of our ministers visited, and that the doctor on call was a member of the church, as was the chaplain who visited our room and blessed the tiny body I couldn't bring myself to hold. We were embraced by our community before we even knew them.

In the bleakness of the days to come, though, I lost sight of God. I lost that holiness. We were sent home within hours of our arrival, empty-handed, empty-hearted, empty-wombed. With bitterness and anger, I dealt with the aftermath in the next days and weeks—an aching body, breasts engorged with no one to feed, ashes and tiny inked footprints for which we still have no right place, and the onslaught of compassionate but awful platitudes. I didn't talk about it, because there were no words. I cried myself dry and sobbed myself sick.

Where is God in this?

I know the "right" answers, but I cannot yet believe them. I know that God suffers in our suffering. I know that God does not leave us, that there is nowhere we can go that God cannot find us. But in those days, and occasionally still in these days, God not only failed to answer my prayers for comfort and peace; God did not even show up to listen.

No, it was not "worth it." I am still angry. I try not to dwell entirely on the ways in which I experienced God's ugly absence. I still want an answer, even as I know that there is none. The grief cannot be unraveled; it can only be enfolded into my story. The crookedness of four awful losses is not set straight by the birth of a daughter. What is lacking is still missed.

We move forward with love, for each other and for this new life entrusted to us, chirping in the next room even as I write. I feel my way back into faith, back into hope. I open my heart to receive God's grace.

I don't forget.

## Prayer

Holy God, help us to feel your presence even in the emptiness, and your grace even in what seems like the most profound absence. Be with us in the awful stillness, and speak to us through the dreadful silence. Hold us, your grieving daughters and sons, and do not let the pain, the anger, and the sorrow overwhelm our lives. Amen.

> **Stephanie McLeskey** is a university chaplain affiliated with the Cooperative Baptist Fellowship, living and working in Mars Hill, North Carolina. She grew up in and around Atlanta, Georgia, and attended Candler School of Theology at Emory University. She and her husband, Ken, are members of First Baptist Church of Asheville.

# God Never Left

## Rachel Whaley Doll

In the depths of infertility, I desperately searched the Bible for Light in my darkness. I connected with Job for a while, until I got to the "happy ending" where "the Lord restored the fortunes of Job" (Job 42:10). It felt like the lives of his wife and the children lost were not important, and this made me angrier. Every instance of infertility in the Bible ended with "God opened her womb," as if God had closed it in the first place. I will never understand why infertility was part of my journey, but I know that the God that loves me and created me did not orchestrate that hell. After a while, I stopped asking "why?" and simply starting looking for connection.

The Psalms did offer some comfort, because the psalmist seemed to be the only one who was honest about the hard times. I finally found Psalm 139, and took comfort in the fact that it did not say God knows me "because I am worthy" or "because I have made good choices and been nice to everyone." It simply says God knows me, whatever I am feeling, and is with me; even "if I make my bed in Sheol, you are there" (Ps 139:8).

When our sixth round of fertility drugs ended with a miscarriage, I snapped. The anger had been seething in me for so long, and I no longer feared what my "loving" God would do to me if I screamed everything I wanted to say. Once my voice was gone, I sat on the floor for a long time. I think I fell asleep, crumpled on the floor by my bed. I felt something in that moment that has stuck with me.

I had this picture in my head of a waiting room. I had been in there so long that I had grown comfortable in the molded plastic chairs that every hospital waiting room seems to have. Someone was sitting on the floor in the corner, disheveled and tired. Whoever it was would not make eye contact or speak to me. I realized somehow that it was God. I yelled, "Get up! Hold me! Fix this!" But the figure did not move. Eventually my anger subsided enough for me to realize that even though God was not shielding me from this pain, not jumping in and making it right, God never left me alone.

Even when I screamed ugly things and gave up on God, God never left. That disheveled look was God weathering the storm with me. I hold on to that visual when life feels overwhelming and out of control. It's not the picture of God I had when I was a child or, frankly, the picture of God I would choose if I had a choice. But I take strength in knowing that, no matter what, God isn't leaving me. God isn't leaving you, either—no matter where you are or where you are going.

"Where can I go from your spirit? Or where can I flee from your presence? If I ascend to heaven, you are there; if I make my bed in Sheol, you are there" (Ps 139:7-8).

## Prayer

Powerful, Silent Friend, when I have no words, you are there. When I am full of anger and ready to lash out, you are still there. Help me connect with the Light I see in my days, even when it feels dark inside. Remind me again that you will not leave me alone. Amen.

**Rachel Whaley Doll** is an author, biblical storyteller, and Christian educator living in eastern North Carolina. Her latest book is *Beating on the Chest of God: A Faith Journey through Infertility*. Rachel's blog is at rachelwhaleydoll.com.

# In the Wilderness

## Pam Durso

> *Now Sarah, Abram's wife, bore him no children. She had an Egyptian slave-girl whose name was Hagar, and Sarah said to Abram, "You see that the* Lord *has prevented me from bearing children; go in to my slave-girl; it may be that I shall obtain children by her." And Abram listened to the voice of Sarah.* (Genesis 16:1-2)

I remember all too clearly the day we "found out." I remember exactly where we were when we heard the news, and it was not good. We were told that there was a remote possibility, at best, that biological children would be part of our future. Keith and I were just months away from getting married when we got that phone call. When I think about that day, even now, twenty-seven years later, the pain and tears sometimes rush back to greet me just as they did the first time I heard the news. Infertility was a very real and painful threat to my hopes and dreams of becoming a parent, and I was left feeling vulnerable, angry, and confused.

My experience has shaped so many parts of my life, including my reading of Scripture. I find myself drawn to biblical texts that feature "barren" women, and there seem to be a disproportional number of women struggling with infertility in the Old Testament. So many Hebrew women knew, like me, what it was like to live with the pain of not being able to have a child.

Genesis 16 tells the story of one such woman. In this chapter of Genesis, Sarah, the wife of Abraham, is a woman still without a child. She is living in a wilderness, empty and alone, and there seems to be no one who can bring her comfort or end her misery. Even God seems far away, for the promises that God made to her husband about their having a son are still unfulfilled. I can just imagine the questions Sarah asked: Where is this child? Will there ever really be a baby?

Instead of a baby, Sarah has a marriage that is tense and unsettled, and her relationship with God is full of unspoken anger and resentment. Living with that kind of pain and hurt can drive a person to words of desperation, and in Genesis 16:2, we find Sarah crying out. She confronts her husband and says, "The LORD has kept me from having children."

Sarah lays the blame for her infertility fully on God—she believes it is God who has closed her womb, prevented her from conceiving, and she screams out her pain, verbalizing her feelings of abandonment. God has left her. God has turned against her. This God who had made grand promises has not fulfilled any of those promises.

There is a second woman in this story—Hagar. Genesis 16 tells us that Hagar was forced into a sexual relationship with Abraham and told that she must conceive, she must have a baby, she must be a mother, but the baby would not be her own. It would belong to Sarah. Hagar would simply be a surrogate. Abraham and Sarah would use her body. They would use her womb. They would take her child. She had no say.

The rest of the story is not a pretty one. These two hurting women—both alone, both grieving the loss of something they valued—are now swept up in a complicated relationship. Their story is not resolved in these verses or even in this chapter. There is more to come—and it is a complex, chaotic future ahead for all involved. But we know how the story ends. Eventually, Sarah becomes pregnant, and in Genesis 21, we are told of the birth of her son.

Yet it is the Sarah of Genesis 2 that speaks loudest to me, this vulnerable, brokenhearted Sarah who is desperately searching for relief from grief, heartache, and loss. Knowing the Sarah of Genesis 2 and knowing the end of her story tells me this: while she may have felt that God was far away from her, God was in reality always with her, even in her deepest grief, even in her loneliest wilderness, even when she used and abused another in a desperate attempt to have a baby. Even at her lowest moment, God did not turn away from or desert her—even as she turned against God, God was there.

This story offers me assurance that in my moments of deepest pain, in my times of greatest vulnerability, on my darkest days, I can cry out in honesty to God. I can take my questions, my anger, and my pain and speak them aloud to God. I don't have to mask my feelings or hide my hostility. I can scream out even as Sarah did, "The LORD has caused this."

And I can rest in the knowledge that God is there. God is there in the shadows of my life, in my darkest places, in my wilderness. God is there when I feel alone. God is there in my despair. Even when I cannot trust God, even when I cannot sense God's presence, even when I blame God for the injustices of life, God never turns away. God is with me.

## Prayer

In the shadows of my life, in my darkest places, in my wilderness, O God, you are there. Open my eyes to see you. Open my heart to sense your presence. Open my soul to receive your spirit. Amen.

> **Pam Durso** is the executive director of Baptist Women in Ministry, an independent Baptist organization that supports and advocates for Baptist women ministers. She loves walking alongside and encouraging women called by God to ministry. Pam also enjoys researching, writing, and teaching in the area of Baptist history. She teaches Baptist history as an adjunct professor at McAfee School of Theology. She and her husband, Keith, live in Lawrenceville, Georgia, with their son, Michael, and daughter, Alex.

# Redemption in the Dark

## Rebekah McLeod Hutto

> *The light shines in the darkness, and the darkness did not overcome it.* (John 1:5)

I told the members of my church that God and I were having some quiet time. Borrowing this quote from a friend, I let them in on a secret: my relationship with God is too important to let the death of our baby girl go unnoticed. I was holding God to account, and I needed some healing to take place in order for conversation between the two of us to resume. God and I had some quiet time for many weeks. I won't say that I've experienced complete healing as of this writing, but God and I are at least back on speaking terms.

One of the reasons we're talking again is that I've realized that, although we promote a light-infused God in our theology, God does some pretty amazing work in the dark as well. The dark is where I've found myself since losing my daughter at twenty weeks. I have felt lost because my flashlight of faith, so to speak, is no longer big enough to see or predict my and my family's future. After having the ground collapse beneath us, we have no idea what's next. I've suffered miscarriage before, but the loss of the baby girl I was coming to know and feel in my second trimester ripped me to the core.

Moreover, there's no rhyme or reason why it all happened, why my water broke, and why I couldn't save her. Renaming this darkness as "trauma" has helped with the nightmares and intense anxiety I faced in the months afterward. But even though I'm in a physically healthier place now, the world continues to feel dark. How do we trust that we won't be traumatized again by another tragedy, not to mention future pregnancies? Even though I know and believe in the love of Christ, I've struggled to find the light in the darkness that John speaks of in his Gospel. Lately, putting one foot in front of the other feels like stepping into the cold unknown, and I'm grasping for some sort of direction.

Coincidentally, a favorite author and theologian came to my rescue. I've been reading Barbara Brown Taylor's new book, *Learning to Walk in the Dark*, and she's helping me see that God's presence is not always about the light. The above Scripture text from the Gospel of John is comforting, and many have spoken these words to me in order to help me make sense of our dark tragedy. But in my desperate search for light and direction in the months afterward, I forgot something about our God: even if the darkness seems to overcome us, God is just as present there as in the light. Taylor has challenged me to ask myself, "If Christ is already sitting with me in the dark, why am I so eager to turn on the light?"

God took Abraham out at night to count the stars, God wrestled with and blessed Jacob in the middle of the night, manna fell from heaven before morning, and God spoke to Moses and the people from a cloud of darkness. And finally, in that cold, empty, and dark tomb, Christ gave life to the most depressed place we've ever known: the resurrection happened in the darkness of a cave.

There is redemption in the dark. Taylor is reminding me to seek God in the darkest places of my soul and find that there is life even when the lights go out, and possibly even more when we can't find a light to turn on. Faith in the midst of tragedy is not about sentimental gestures of hope. Mine is about sitting with God in the dark, trusting that wisdom and guidance can be found in the quiet, lonely, lights out, nighttime places of faith.

## *Prayer*

Ever loving and caring God, we come before you, humbled by the mysteries of life and death. Help us to accept what we cannot understand, to have faith where reason fails, to have courage in the midst of disappointment. Help us to remember that you breathe life into the depths of our dark despair. In the strong name of Jesus, we pray, Amen.

**Rebekah McLeod Hutto** is a Presbyterian (USA) pastor and Associate Minister of Christian Education and Discipleship at Brick Presbyterian Church in New York City. Originally from Greenville, South Carolina, Rebekah is serving her second call in ordained ministry at Brick and married to B. J. Hutto, also an ordained pastor. They live in New York City with their daughter, Hannah Ruth.

# Light Shines in the Darkness: We Are Not Alone

# Grief Changes

## Mary Elizabeth Hill Hanchey

*It is my grief that the right hand of the Most High has changed.* (Psalm 77:10)

Your grief will change. Though it has seemed too heavy a burden to bear, though it has been so bulky, so intrusive, that it has been hard to imagine living a full life with this grief in tow, it will change. It will not go away, but it will become something that you are able to carry around with you. You will be able to pack it up. It will not always saturate everything that you do.

For years, this has been the hope that I offer to those who are struggling under the heavy burden of fertility grief—whose infertility brings pain again and again and again; whose abrupt loss of a pregnancy shatters a peaceful dream of things to come; whose loss of a new baby crushes their hope and their heart so that even breathing seems too difficult a task.

I know this because I bear witness to the change that has taken place in the grief of my peers who have lost and gone on to have more children. I know this because I bear witness to the change that has taken place in the grief of my peers who have lost and have never had more children, whose lives have unfolded down paths that could never have been guessed. I know this because my own grief has changed.

The grief I carry with me is complicated. There were two miscarriages interspersed with the births of healthy children who could not have been mine had I not lost the others. But they are not replacements. They are simply my children. And then there was the birth of a child who nearly died the day she was born and then several times afterward, who fought with truly supernatural strength to overcome bizarre medical emergencies, and who lived. She is a miracle. But her life does not erase the long, dark nights when we did not know whether she would ever leave the hospital, and when we struggled to find the light in our darkness.

Those griefs still take up space in my being. They are not in danger of evaporating on this side of life. But that is reasonable. There is enough space in my being for them. They do not keep me from moving forward.

I was doing a lectio divina reading of Psalm 77 (NRSV) with other women who are tangled in fertility grief when I heard my friend say these words: "It is my grief that the right hand of the Most High has changed." I was startled. I had been saying that for years, but the psalmist declares it? And the psalmist declares it just after railing about the Lord spurning and forgetting to be gracious and shutting up compassion (Ps 77:7-9, NRSV).

This claim is our promise. The changing of our grief does not depend on our own right thinking. We join a great cloud of witnesses whose railing against God is their only acknowledgment that God even exists. And in so doing, we are part of a great cloud of witnesses who will one day join the psalmist in declaring, "It is my grief that the right hand of the Most High has changed" (Ps 77:10, NRSV).

## Prayer

God in whom we live and grieve and have our very being, change our grief! Grab hold of us and turn the deluge of weeping into a spring of life; turn our rage into energy for walking and breathing; turn our writhing into embrace so that we might shelter those whose grief is more raw; breathe your spirit into the crevices of our being to make space for the grief that will be our companion. So may it be.

**Mary Elizabeth Hill Hanchey** lives with her family in Durham, North Carolina, where she is a member of Watts Street Baptist Church, a part of the Hannah Ministry planning team, and co-founder of Project Pomegranate. She holds a JD from UNC-Chapel Hill and is completing an MDiv at Duke Divinity School.

# Expecting

## Holly Jarrell-Marcinelli

*Come Thou long-expected Jesus,*
*Born to set Thy people free;*
*From our fears and sins release us;*
*Let us find our rest in Thee.*
*Israel's strength and consolation,*
*Hope of all the earth Thou art;*
*Dear desire of every nation,*
*Joy of every longing heart.* (Charles Wesley, 1744)

As I write this, it is Advent, a season when we join together to wait with a frightened but faithful young virgin and centuries of Christians for the arrival of a very special baby. Every year we wait until we nearly burst with anticipation, until that warm and glorious moment when we celebrate—the baby is here! We crowd around a feeding trough in a dirty shed to peer at this infant, this improbable, helpless creature who has been sent to save us.

I love Advent. It is my favorite season of the church year. As a child, I was the one in my family *not* begging to open a present or two early, on Christmas Eve. I preferred to wait until Christmas Day, to let the anticipation build. Back then, it's true, I loved the "expecting." But the idea of "expecting" is different for me now.

During the preceding spring, my husband and I underwent another IVF procedure, and I got pregnant. It was perfect. Our first round back in the infertility ring after our daughter's birth eighteen months earlier was a success, and I was relieved that it appeared our fertility struggles would not be as prolonged the second time around. Our baby was to be born around Christmas—around now.

Heartbreakingly, I lost the pregnancy very early. But in the ensuing months, I haven't forgotten the timeline that would have been had I continued to live out my ritual of expecting. I would have tried to hide my morning sickness during that busy and demanding period at work in May and June. We would have announced the good news to our friends at our annual summer gathering in July. I would have worn a maternity dress to the fall weddings we attended. We would have been transitioning our now two-year-old out of her crib and into a bed to make room for her younger sibling.

And here, in these Advent days, I would have felt a kinship with my sister Mary in the moments when I sat with my hand on my belly, feeling the gentle nudges and dances within. Together, across the centuries, we sisters would wait, and our waiting would radiate with joy, with love, with hope.

Those who are struggling with infertility know well the meaning of the phrase "long expected," particularly the "long" part. What we wouldn't give to be "expecting" for ourselves this season. Our life is taken over by our "dear desire," and we understand deeply what it means to have a "longing heart" beat within our chest. Charles Wesley's gift to us in the poetry of this hymn is his reminder of the Hope within the expecting. This exercise does not hold only uncertainty and exhaustion. Jesus will be our strength to forge ahead on the journey, and our consolation when the pain is raw and the emptiness sounds thunderous echoes in our hearts.

The word "consolation," in this hymn, is the poetic balm to our wounds. The "sole" part of "console" comes from a Latin word meaning "to comfort" (it is the same word from which our "solace" is derived). But solace and comfort can fall short when offered from a distance, a gift dropped off at the door and left for us to unpack on our own. The healing power of the word "consolation" comes from the "con-," a Latin root meaning "with" or "together." Israel's "consolation" sits in the depths of our sorrow with us, does not stain the silence with empty assurances, joins in our song of weary sadness, and remains with us long after the others have gone.

Expecting is so much more than waiting. It is waiting with hope and confidence in the outcome. Often, hope is too much for us to carry on our own, especially for such a long journey, and we need others to help us. When I initially told some of my friends that we would be trying IVF to get pregnant, I was repeatedly taken aback by their reactions of excitement for us. How could they feel excited?

I was not excited about the challenges that lay ahead, but I came to understand that my friends were seeing beyond those short-term challenges. They had a vision of what was to come, and they were carrying the hope for me when I could not. God has given us many promises and reasons to hope. With God as my companion, I can embrace the expecting, long as it may be.

## Prayer

God, you are the great Consolation who will never leave me to wait alone. Release me, oh Comforter, from my fears of failure, loneliness, and disappointment, and from my sins of faithlessness, bitterness, and resentment. My desire and my joy, let me find my rest in Thee. Amen.

> **Holly Jarrell-Marcinelli** attends Christ Church (Episcopal) in Andover, Massachusetts, where she serves as a verger, eucharistic minister, and a member of the Altar Guild. Holly is a licensed social worker, specializing in geriatric social work.

# A Shared Hope

## Deborah Gaddis Reeves

> *Now faith is the assurance of things hoped for, the conviction of things not seen.* (Hebrews 11:1)

As a child at play, I preferred most often to pretend I was a mother. I carried a doll on my hip and a diaper bag on my shoulder almost anywhere. I imagined myself a mom. Though my responses when asked what I wanted to "be" when I grow up changed many times, the dream that remained constantly in my mind was motherhood. Loving adults in my life assured me that I could be anything I wanted to be when I grew up. I knew I would be a mother someday.

My professional journey led me to full-time ministry, to ordination, and ultimately to chaplaincy in health-care settings. As a hospital chaplain, I was invited into the sacred and devastating spaces of ectopic pregnancies, miscarriages, stillborn births, and infant deaths. I participated in the blessing, anointing, and baptism of these precious babies in the midst of the darkest grief.

Along the journey, I learned of the miraculous nature of every new life. It is not as easy to conceive and bear a healthy baby as I once was warned in sex-education class. When my husband and I started dating years ago, his mother asked me if I would have children someday. My response was, "I hope I am able." She asked if there was a reason I may not be able. Recalling the many parents with whom I journeyed in the depths of despair, and remembering that there most often is not an explanation, reason, or understanding of such loss, I knew that her question was not an easy one to answer. Informed by nothing except experience, I simply answered, "I don't know." Ironies sometimes are cruel. The experiences that informed a response to my mother in-law's question have now become my own. I still imagine myself a mom. I no longer *know* that I will be a mother someday. I just hope.

With hope comes disappointment, doubt, and grief. When my husband and I were diagnosed with unexplained infertility, he asserted that we still have hope since the fertility specialists were unable to identify a reason we could not conceive. Together we hoped. When we later miscarried after a successful intrauterine insemination, our doctor asserted that we still have hope because the miscarriage indicated that conception is possible. That certainly is a scientific way of coping with such a loss, but my husband and I grieved individually and together. Hope became more and more difficult to muster. We decided to acknowledge the significance of this loss of life by sharing it with our family, trusted friends, and members of our church. For years, we had wandered in the desert of infertility practically alone. Making our grief journey known was an important step in bearing light to the darkness.

In hearing our story, people responded by telling their own stories of grief, loss, hope, and success associated with infertility. My husband and I listened to the stories of couples experiencing similar grief, journeying the wilderness together. Other people shared encouraging stories that culminated in miraculous conception, adoption, foster parenting, or newfound meaning and fulfillment in caring for nieces, nephews, or other children in their communities. In sharing, hope was nurtured.

My husband and I continue to journey with both hope and doubt. Though I so often pray eloquently for others in their times of despair, the only words I seem to find when speaking to God on my behalf are "Please, Lord, please." The details of what I am asking are no longer clear to me. I hope in a desire that sometimes is unimaginable. I try not to doubt, and I always try to hope. Though I cannot be sure I will be a mother, this journey requires such childlike faith, the belief in things not seen.

One couple who shared their story with us ultimately was blessed with a successful pregnancy through in-vitro fertilization. I cried tears of joy through the service of dedication in which our church celebrated the life of this miracle baby named Mason. When the pastor asked the congregation what is our promise to this child, we read responsively, proclaiming that we will teach him about Abraham and

Sarah, the grandparents of our faith. In that moment, I realized that the very couple with whom our faith originates knew the pain of a barren womb. Ironies sometimes are beautiful. Mason, the child whose name means "stone-layer," is a reminder to me of a faith built on the foundation of *hope for a child*. Though grief and doubt are ever present, hope is nurtured when the journey is shared with others. It is a journey in faith. "Now faith is the assurance of things hoped for, the conviction of things not seen" (Heb 11:1, NRSV).

## Prayer

Please, Lord, please.
Help my unbelief.
Please, Lord, please.
Nurture my faith in things unseen.
Please, Lord, please.
Accept my gratitude for others who journey with me in grief, in disappointment, in doubt, and in hope.
Please, Lord, please.
Make your presence known in this darkness.
Please, Lord, please.
Bear light to my longing for, to my aching for, to my asking for, and to my hoping for a promise of the newness of life.
Please, Lord, please.
Create within me such a promise.
Please, Lord, please.
Grant me this desire of my heart, Divine Creator and God of Love.
Please, Lord, please.
In the name of your Son, I pray: please, Lord, please.
Amen.

**Deborah Gaddis Reeves** is originally from North Carolina. Deborah met Stephen Reeves, a native Texan, at a conference on social justice. They were married in 2008. Deborah and Stephen currently live in Georgia, having relocated recently from their home in Texas. Their church membership remains with First Baptist Church in Austin. Deborah is a graduate of the University of North Carolina at Chapel Hill, and the School of Divinity at Gardner-Webb University. She has served as a minister to children and families at a church in North Carolina, as a chaplain to disaster survivors in Mississippi and Louisiana, as a hospital chaplain in North Carolina and Texas, and most recently as a hospice chaplain for Hospice Austin. Deborah was ordained by Boiling Springs Baptist Church in North Carolina and is endorsed by the Cooperative Baptist Fellowship. She is a board-certified chaplain through Board of Chaplaincy Certification, Inc., and is a member of the Association of Professional Chaplains.

# Deeply Marked

## Elise Erikson Barrett

> *But Zion said, "The Lord has forsaken me,*
> *my Lord has forgotten me."*
> *Can a woman forget her nursing child,*
> *or show no compassion for the child of her womb?*
> *Even these may forget,*
> *yet I will not forget you.*
> *See, I have inscribed you on the palms of my*
> *hands . . . .* (Isaiah 49:14-16a)

Weeks after our first miscarriage, which had begun during worship in a trickle of blood and rushed from my body in the days after like a flood I bore with me, I sat on the floor of the house we rented, a divinity school student longing to love God again. I dug my fingers into matted shag carpeting, tried and failed to pray in the early morning stillness. The news that we were invading Iraq had just spilled out of the alarm clock radio speakers, and I sat, the membrane between the global pain outside of me and the deepening pain within me feeling at risk of dissolution.

    I did not trust God. I did not trust God to care for this lost little one, this stirring within me that had been more spark than flame, more seed than sturdy plant, more potentiality than fulfillment. She had been fragile, dependent on my body to protect and nourish her until her lungs could handle the rush of air, until her heart could beat surrounded by her body, until her eyes were lidded and could hold the light. Something . . . A hormone? A chemical? A chromosomal splitting gone awry? Who could know, but something had gone wrong and she was gone and I had failed, or God had failed, or the brokenness of the world had made itself known in the dark mystery of my body, and what was vulnerable had been expelled and died in a trickle and a flood of helpless bleeding. And I wrapped myself around the pain because I did not want her forgotten as well as failed.

And to hold the grief I made a tough-boundaried space in myself, a leathery egg, heavy and opaque.

It was heavy, but it was substantial, and its weight comforted me even as my heart ached with it.

Months later, in a memorial service created and led by the members of my clinical pastoral education group, I sat again, feeling untouched and almost irritated by the absurdity of worship centered on a pregnancy loss half a year ago, distanced from God, nursing the leaden weight I continued to carry.

And then the preacher, all shiny red hair and compassion, looked straight at me and said, "Elise, what is found in God can never be lost."

I felt the truth of this, and remembered the passage from Isaiah 49. The membranes all dissolved, and the grief poured through me in a flood and lit up translucent to the light and love that God would not let me deny any longer. And I thought that day—and again in later years when we lost more pregnancies, and then again when I held babies that had been pulled through the incision repeated low across my belly—I thought about the way that my body and heart and soul bear the marks of love. Not just generally, but in particular ways, each of our seven pregnancies—the three that brought forth seeds that sprout and grow visibly each day, and the four that ended before I could see the forming bodies—each one marked me. Each life is written in the lines on my hands and furrows across my forehead, the stretch marks on my hips and scars across my belly. I will forget none of them.

And God, who holds my promise and my potential as well as my present, who will love me no more as a wiser, fuller, more fully realized old woman than I am loved today, bears on divine hands the marks of the short living of our lost little ones. Holds in fullness promises that are left unrealized.

We sometimes feel forgotten. We fear we have been forsaken. And then we remember how much we, with our limited love, have compassion for the children of our wombs: the ones for whom we long, the ones we lose, the ones we bear toward their fulfillment. How deeply we are marked by their living and by their dying.

We can trust that our love, our grief, our longing is a reflection of the greater love, grief, and longing of our God. God will not forget. The names of God's children have forever marked God's tender hands.

## Prayer

My God, the storms of loss and grief can threaten my confidence in your love. Remind me that you do not stand far off. Remind me that you have come as close as my tears, as close as my bitterness, as close as my confusion. Remind me that even now, you are holding me close, and my life is being written into your hands. Give me the manna I need to walk one day, and then another, until my wounds are healed and my scars are left to tell the story of faithful love. Amen.

**Elise Erikson Barrett** is a United Methodist pastor, writer, editor, and singer/songwriter living in Spartanburg, South Carolina, with her husband and three children. She is the author of *What Was Lost: A Christian Journey through Miscarriage* (WJK Books, 2010), which was named *Christianity Today*'s "Best Book of 2011" in the Christian Living category. You are warmly invited to connect with Elise through her website, www.elisebarrett.com.

# Where Does My Help Come From?

## Brittany Rasmussen Mackey

> *I lift up my eyes to the hills—from where will my help come? My help comes from the* Lord, *who made heaven and earth.* (Psalm 121:1-2)

While I knew it would take a village to raise a child, I had no idea it would take a village to *make* a child.

Shortly after my husband and I first started trying to get pregnant, it became apparent that it was not going to happen "naturally." We began walking the road of infertility. It was never an easy road, but it was also a road that I never walked alone, even though there were days when I felt lonely.

My village for conception included an obstetrician, a team of fertility specialists, a nutritionist, a pharmacist, an acupuncturist, a massage therapist, a perinatologist, a group of amazingly supportive friends, my family, and my husband. During the times of uncertainty, where did my help come from? My help came from the minds, hearts, and hands of so many people.

I grieved many losses, some real and some perceived, during this journey. I grieved my dreams of motherhood. While my story contains many happy chapters, I did not know while in the midst of the struggle that those chapters would come. I only knew that the raw grief was real, that it was painful, and that it created a sense of betrayal by my own body. During this grief, where did my help come from? My help came from the words, both written and spoken, of people who understood—people who had walked this journey before or people who simply knew what to say.

Community, then, was my help. A community of minds, hearts, and hands, of understanding and supportive words—both written and spoken—sustained me, sustained us. Healed us.

Significantly, though my community of friends and family loved me well, it was an online community—a community of strangers—who supported me the best. Close friends and family, though they wanted to help, often unintentionally tossed out platitudes. But in this virtual community of those who had walked a journey similar to mine, I found friends who listened, spoke when it was helpful, and encouraged me to speak. During this time of potential isolation, where did my help come from? My help came from a healing community of others who walked with me. I was able to experience the healing power of community repeatedly, a lesson that carried over into an extended NICU stay for my twins after they were born at twenty-nine weeks.

Though I found myself supported by relationships with those who understood my grief and frustration, I still had to deal with my relationship with God. Many days I was angry at God and asked, *"Why me?"* I had lived a good life, made good choices, followed the plan I believed God would have me do. I shed lots of tears. Often I found myself crying—for myself, for the loss I felt, or for fear of the unknown. In the midst of the tears and the heartache, this remained true: God loved me, God loved my dream to become a mother, and God loved the children I would eventually come to know and love myself. During this time of immense sadness, where did my help come from? My help came from God, the Creator of life who was sustaining me.

And then came the waiting! Engaged with a supportive virtual community, living in God's love, I still faced excruciating waiting. The waiting between bloodwork, between ultrasounds, between phone calls from doctors, between monthly periods, between the next steps, whatever that would be.

While it was not easy, over time I learned what to do during the waiting. I continued to live my life. I learned to live in the moment, but instead of living in fear, loss, guilt, or sadness I learned to live with hope and anticipation of the future, no matter what that looked like. Of course, it was not easy, but it was possible. During this time of immeasurable waiting, where did my help come from? My help came from the distraction of the daily ritual of living.

This was, perhaps, the most helpful way for friends and family who did not know what to say—they kept me busy. What used to seem very ordinary became my refuge from the monotony of trying to get pregnant medically.

The infertility journey is never easy, and so mine was not. I did not walk that journey with as much grace as I wished for. I limped around with what little energy I could muster. I often felt as I though I suffered in silence, but I found my voice and learned to share my story.

During that season of longing, I learned to be patient and to wait on the promises God had for my family and for me. My emotional baggage was heavy and filled with sadness, loneliness, jealousy, guilt, anger, betrayal, hurt, disappointment, and denial, yet never in my life had I felt God's promises so strongly.

For me, pregnancy would never be just something that happened; it would never be unplanned; it would never be taken for granted. For me, it would be so much more. It would be fulfillment of a dream and completion of a journey.

## Prayer

God, the maker and lover of all life, be and bring help to all of those who seek it. Where there is isolation, gather community. Where there are hurtful words, bring quiet. Where there is doubt and anger and fear, bring a deep realization of Your love. Where there is waiting, provide ritual and activity to occupy the fretful mind. Amen.

**Brittany Rasmussen Mackey** has an undergraduate degree in Elementary Education and a master's degree in Urban Policy Studies. She has lived and worked in Atlanta, Georgia, for thirteen years as a teacher, a non-profit director, and currently as a full-time mom to three amazing daughters.

# Knowing You in My Heart

## Susan A. Joyce

*My frame was not hidden from you, when I was being made in secret, intricately woven in the depths of the earth.* (Psalm 139:15, NRSV)

Known but not seen. Loved but not touched. The child I lost was known and loved but never seen and never touched. How is it that we can know someone and yet never lay eyes on him or her? And how can we love someone so deeply without sharing a relationship, other than to know that the tiny one is somehow a part of us, moving and growing and becoming? To grieve for something that has not yet become is inexplicable, but all the time we grieve for dreams not realized, for hopes that have not come to fruition.

Scripture teaches us that God loved us even before our frames were knitted together, before we had become, before our lives were realized. As much as I loved my little being yet to be, the new life that was to be ours, God loved that life, too. As I imagined tiny fingers and hands, innocent smiles and gurgling coos, God had already seen and heard.

The child I never saw, I knew in my heart. While fingers and toes had not time to develop before the child was gone, that life was there, growing. I had only begun to feel the flutters when they vanished, but the life was there, growing. I knew it was there before the doctor confirmed it. And yet, within weeks, all the dreams and plans and excitement turned into painful waiting, and finally loss, as life and blood and water emptied itself from a protective womb. Blood and water could be replenished, but not that life. I could not wrap my arms around that little life, but God could, and did.

At first I rationalized: *I already have three children. They are healthy and thriving. This pain is a part of life.* But the sadness would not go away. The feeling of loss could not be dismissed. The emptiness in my womb and in my heart was certain.

As much as I wanted my husband to understand, he had not carried this life, had not known this life, had not loved this life in the ways that I had. His support and love meant much, but my pain sought expression and understanding, and so my words became silent prayers spoken to the One who had known and loved this life like I had. I had questions with no answers, pain with no words, emptiness with no solace, faith with no understanding.

From time to time, I wonder what it would have been like for this child to be living, to be a real part of our family, to be known even as I knew, to be loved even as I had loved. But those are matters to be settled in eternity. Then, as now, I can only surrender to the heart of the One who knew my frame before it was knitted together, and who still holds the frame of this precious life, until one day we no longer see through the glass darkly, and we know even as we are known. On that day we will see face to face, heart to heart, and God will introduce me to the child I have never seen.

## *Prayer*

Holy God who knows us, our frames, our minds, our desires, and our journeys, hold us in our grief, in our deepness calling to your deepness, as we search for understanding of the painful events in our lives. You, the author of hopes and dreams, the giver of life, hold us when dreams are shattered and life interrupted. You, the first and the last, help us to trust in your wisdom and love and grace, that as much as you hold the world together, you hold each of us, moving in our lives and moving in this world, to bring us to a time when we can hope and love and laugh again. We pray in the name of Christ, Amen.

**Susan A. Joyce** was born in Petersburg, Virginia, and received her Bachelor of Science in Mathematics from the College of William and Mary in Williamsburg, where she met her husband, Christopher Joyce. They have three sons, Peyton, Justin, and Collin, and two daughters-in-law, Rachelle and Christy. Reverend Joyce has worked a multitude of different jobs, including mothering and volunteering for anything and everything while her children were growing up. Shortly after a move to Farmville, Virginia, she sensed God calling her to full-time ministry, and in 1999 she was ordained to the gospel ministry by Farmville Baptist Church. She earned her Master of Divinity in 2005 from the Baptist Theological Seminary at Richmond and in 2006 answered a call to Antioch Baptist Church in Enfield, North Carolina, where she currently serves as pastor.

# I Believe

## KATIE ROSCOE

> *Immediately the father of the child cried out, "I believe; help my unbelief!"* (Mark 9:24)

The father was tired. He had watched his son suffer for so long. This boy was the light of his life, the apple of his eye, his very heart. He had such dreams for his son. And then the suffering began. His son writhed and convulsed, uncontrolled and uncontrollable. His father had rescued him when the fits threw him into dangerous places, but he could not rescue his child from the torment that plagued him. He had tried everything; nothing worked. But someone told them about Jesus. Jesus . . . the man from Galilee who spoke of the kingdom of heaven, who claimed God as his Father, who healed the sick. The father brought his son to Jesus. Would Jesus even notice them? The crowd was so large. The disciples met them first. They tried to heal the boy, but they could not do it. They seemed perplexed and puzzled at their inability to cast the evil spirit out. But then Jesus saw them. The father, in a rush of emotion, began to tell his son's story. He looked at Jesus and cried in desperation, "If you are able, take pity on us and help us!"

Jesus looked at him. His eyes were kind as he responded, "If you are able? All things can be done for the one who believes." The father felt hope for the first time in years. "I believe," he cried. "Help my unbelief!"

I believe, too . . . but I need help when life shakes my faith and my doubts surface. After two miscarriages, I was tired. But we were excited and hopeful when I found out I was pregnant again. We heard our baby's heartbeat and saw her little body on the screen! We faithfully filled out our new pregnancy journal. But then things started going wrong.

As I lay in bed and prayed, I cried out in desperation to God. "Lord, you can save our baby. You can! I believe in your power. Please,

God, save our baby." But these questions stayed with me: What if God didn't do what I wanted? What if we lost another baby? What then? My body and heart were so tired that I felt my faith falter. Would I be able to believe if the prayers I had prayed and the hope that I had placed in God didn't make things turn out the way I wanted?

I lost that baby. The grief was nearly debilitating. I couldn't understand. But in the midst of the pain God came closer. In a way that I can't fully explain, I felt the presence of God holding me close. Even in the moments when I cried out in anger and the times when I was so numb I didn't want to pray, God held me. I felt God in the arms of my husband as he held me close, in the tears of those who cried with us, and in the moments of stillness and peace that swept over me. And I was reminded that the babies we had lost were in the presence of God.

I couldn't understand why God didn't intervene and save our baby. But in the darkness of that time I learned to believe in a deeper way. I learned that God does not have to answer my prayers the way that I want in order for me to love and trust God. I learned that God loves me even when I have trouble believing and even when God doesn't give me what I ask for.

God loves us. God loves our children, those we hold and treasure and those we never meet face to face. God hears the cries of anguished parents whose hearts beat for their little ones. We are God's precious children, the ones he sent his beloved Son, Jesus, to redeem, and God knows our hurts and holds us close. God hears our prayers and carries us when we cannot believe. God helps us to believe. Thanks be to God.

## *Prayer*

Dear God, thank you for loving us so much that you carry us through the dark and difficult days. Thank you for holding us close when we struggle and for promising us a future that is good and joyful. Thank you for the tears you allow us to cry and for wiping them away as you heal our pain. Help us to keep believing. In Jesus' name I pray, Amen.

**Katie Roscoe** is a South Carolina native with a BA from Columbia College and an MDiv from McAfee School of Theology. She has served churches in Atlanta, Columbia, and, most recently, Southern Pines, North Carolina. Currently, Katie is grateful to be a stay-at-home mom. She is married to John, and they have one son and two noisy dogs! They enjoy living in Pinehurst, North Carolina.

# When I Was a Desolate Woman

ANONYMOUS

*Sing, O barren one who did not bear;*
*burst into song and shout,*
*you who have not been in labor!*
*For the children of the desolate woman will be more*
*than the children of her that is married, says the* LORD.
(Isaiah 54:1, NRSV)

This verse is the first one in Isaiah 54. It speaks to me, though it is a difficult passage. I can recite most of Isaiah 54 by heart because it was the one Scripture that gave me hope during my darkest hour. And my hour was a dark one. The story of my pregnancy and marriage gives my loss another layer. Another texture.

The year started happily for me. I had graduated with my master's degree and met the man of my dreams.

Hoping to be married one day, I had long kept a diary for the man I would marry, a man I had not yet met. I began each entry with "Dear Boaz" and ended it with "Love always, Ruth." I enjoyed sharing my daily adventures, which mostly consisted of writing papers and reading countless articles, with my virtual spouse.

Being a full-time student afforded me little time for dating, so I decided to give online matchmaking a try. What was the worst that could happen? If it didn't work out, I could end my subscription and go back to the old-fashioned way of meeting someone, like running into him at the local supermarket or perhaps at church. I gave online dating a go for a few months but quickly decided that it wasn't for me. It felt superficial and contrived . . . *until* one of my matches mentioned that he was looking for his Ruth. My heart skipped a beat.

I had enough sense to know that I couldn't rely on a single comment from a complete stranger; I had to get to know this guy to make sure he was the one for me. And I was pleasantly surprised. He was a perfect gentleman who worked in the medical field, had a close-knit family, and was a Christian. Check, check, check, and CHECK! After "talking" for several months online, we finally decided to meet face to face. Our courtship was a bit of a whirlwind, and the rest was, as is so often said, history. We got married six months after our first date!

My husband and I had talked about starting a family from the beginning, and it wasn't long before God answered that prayer. We conceived a baby girl a few weeks into our marriage and were absolutely ecstatic. And then it began: our marriage started to fall apart as rapidly as my belly grew. I was miles away from my family, and the one person who had vowed to love me until death grew more distant by the day. After sixteen weeks of going to doctor's appointments alone and reading countless baby books on my own, I guess it was only fitting for me to miscarry without my husband by my side. I was alone.

In less than a year, I lost my husband and my child, as well as my will to live. I was broken. I didn't want to be around other people, and the thought of going to church or reading my Bible seemed counterproductive because of what I chose to believe about God: I was hung up on divorce, on a divorce I had not wanted and that I believed God hated. I felt that God was disappointed with me.

Yet I could not stay away from church, and I could not stay away from the Bible. And, as I was preparing to go to church for the first time after my miscarriage and divorce, I stumbled across this passage in Isaiah.

> Do not fear, for you will not be ashamed;
> do not be discouraged, for you will not suffer disgrace;
> for you will forget the shame of your youth,
> and the disgrace of your widowhood you will remember no more.
> For your Maker is your husband,
> the LORD of hosts is his name;
> the Holy One of Israel is your Redeemer,
> the God of the whole earth he is called. (Isaiah 54:4-5)

I opened my Bible that fateful morning to read a short passage in the book of Psalms but landed here instead. And I'm so glad I did. These verses proved to be my greatest source of strength when I was a desolate woman.

*Prayer*

God, may those who are desolate now learn to sing. May they hear your voice and feel your presence in the midst of this grief. May they know that they are never alone. Amen.

> This author, who writes anonymously, attends a non-denominational church in North Carolina. She works as an advocate for justice issues related to health care.

# When Suffering Gives Birth to Beauty

## Todd Maberry

The biggest challenge that my wife and I have needed to overcome in our marriage was a struggle with infertility that lasted almost five years. Infertility can cause a great amount of suffering, but this suffering can be difficult to understand unless you experience it firsthand. Infertility produces a numbing pain of absence, of nothingness where there should be life.

My wife experienced so much pain and suffering. The suffering was partly mental and emotional. Trips to Target became disasters when walking by the baby section or noticing other pregnant women in the store. Facebook became a source of pain as others posted news of pregnancies and pictures of their infants. The suffering was also physical because her many medications produced terrible side effects. She had several surgeries and countless procedures. Her body gave her monthly reminders that her time had not yet come. Tension arose in our marriage when my level of grief could not match hers. The whole ordeal threatened to consume our minds and thoughts so that we were forgetting why we got married in the first place.

On top of all that, it felt like God was missing and absent. That God did not care about our situation. That we were somehow being punished. After all, we had done all of the right things. We waited until we were married and financially stable before trying to have kids, yet none of that seemed to matter. We lived in an impoverished neighborhood in Durham, North Carolina. While we were struggling and suffering, our neighbor across the street who was hopelessly addicted to crack cocaine became pregnant. Still we waited. Together we shed many tears and cried out to an absent God, "How long?"

And then, in the midst of that suffering, beauty emerged. Both of us discovered strength that we never knew we had. Best of all, friends and family surrounded us with encouragement and support.

Our church family showed us love far beyond what we ever deserved or earned. A primary source of light in that dark time was our friend Monika, who walked beside us so faithfully that we gifted our baby girl with that name when she finally arrived.

In our experience, suffering gave birth to beauty. When I reflect on our struggle with infertility, God *was* present—even though it rarely, if ever, felt like it. God was present through our friends and family who loved us in the hard times. God was present in the strength we did not know we had. The suffering stretched us, and now I see God in our increased ability to experience joy and empathize with those who are suffering.

Even so, it is also important to name the harsh reality that life does not always work out as we wish it would. Despite the scripts that we have all been fed, not all stories have a happy ending. Not all struggles with infertility end with a child. If that is your story, the only hope I can offer in you in this moment is the story of Jesus. The name of Jesus is Emmanuel, which is a word that means "God with us." In Jesus Christ, God became flesh and dwelled among us. Ultimately, Jesus' life was marked by pain and suffering. The night before he was crucified, he wept bitterly and begged God to take away the suffering he knew he would face. He ended up dying on the cross, feeling completely forsaken by a seemingly absent God.

But the story did not end there. The story of Jesus is that absolutely nothing, not even death, is able to keep us from the presence and love of God. If you are in the midst of a time of pain and suffering, I want to encourage you and offer you a word of hope. One of our favorite quotes as we struggled with infertility was from Winston Churchill: "If you are going through hell . . . keep going." Keep going. Do not give up. Start looking for signs of beauty in the midst of the suffering. My hope and my prayer is that if you do look for signs of beauty that are being birthed by your suffering, you will discover that God is present even if you do not feel God's nearness.

## Prayer

God, in those moments of darkness when it feels like you are absent, where are you? How long will I have to be here? What am I supposed to do? Please give me the strength to keep going and the eyes to see the beauty that is being birthed by this suffering. Amen.

> **Todd Maberry** is the Community Pastor at the United Methodist Church of the Resurrection Downtown in Kansas City, Missouri. His wife Laura is a licensed professional counselor working at a private practice in Kansas City. They have a beautiful daughter, Monika, who was born in June 2013. Monika was conceived through a fourth attempt at IVF and after a five-year struggle with infertility.

# Resting My Eyes

## R. P. Fugarino

*And Jesus said to them, "What are you discussing with each other while you walk along?" They stood still, looking sad.* (Luke 24:17)

Our miscarriage was very public. It was also the end to our first pregnancy.

At the time, my wife and I served two different congregations. We had been open about the conception with both of them, and the miscarriage happened on a church mission trip. Because of this, our miscarriage was very public—for better or worse.

In its aftermath, a couple from my congregation asked us what we would have named the child. We told them, and soon after they presented us with a large granite memorial stone engraved with the name we'd shared with them. Such a stone had been meaningful for this couple after a stillbirth, and they wanted to share their tradition with us. We were touched, blessed.

So when the third Sunday in June rolled around, when Father's Day eventually came in for a landing, I had a commemorative stone sitting on my patio, but I did not have a child.

I have never really liked Father's Day. I didn't like it before this experience, and even now with a healthy daughter (seven going on seventeen) seeking to dominate my existence, I still have been slow to come around.

I know it is cliché to say it, but to me Father's Day still feels contrived to sell bourbon, ties, and prime cuts of beef. Besides, don't we procreating guys already get enough days—ample self-congratulatory days of honor on which we watch men and boys mimic war on a football field, days enough to tinker in garages or walk fairways?

So I was pleased when my deep research (ahem, Wikipedia) suggested that America itself was also slow to come around. Apparently, Father's Day as we know it slowly bubbled out of events in

Washington State in early in the twentieth century but was not formally proclaimed until the Johnson administration and then signed into law by Nixon. Some resisted it because of the dogged support given by the likes of tobacco pipe manufacturers.

But a similar and quickly forgotten commemoration happened on July 5, 1908, on the other side of the continent in West Virginia, a few miles from where Mother's Day found its start. It was born out of a woman's grief at her father's death and the shocking deaths of 250 fathers in a nearby mining accident that left 1,000 fatherless children in its wake.

It may sound perverse, and it certainly sounds selfish, but I am a little pleased that at least in a small way, Father's Day itself was brought forth from the soil of loss. After all, the first Father's Day I expected to know as a father became instead a day given to remembering loss.

But I don't think it's perverse, at least not too much. If Easter were just about lilies and sugarcoated marshmallow bunnies, would that be a good thing? But Easter's not just that, of course. It's a shocking, beautiful day born in the shadow of a grave stone, which makes the new life celebrated on Easter that much sweeter and more profound.

So my heart swells a little to know that Father's Day isn't just menswear and sentimentality but also an attempt to combat loss with something beautiful and love-stuffed. For someone who has never cared for the (pseudo)holiday that is Father's Day, that is a remarkable and important development, at least to me.

Anyway, this is certainly on my mind when I take moments to be still in the midst of all of the living that occupies my back patio. I'll hold it especially close on Father's Day when I'll be sitting there sometime in the afternoon. As I sit, I'll have one eye on my daughter as she pesters me about her upcoming birthday party, and my other eye will rest on the stone bearing the name of the child whose birthday party I will never have the opportunity to plan. And I'll take a little comfort in knowing that just a few hours earlier, both of my eyes had been in worship, resting upon the cross on which Jesus died . . . and then rose again.

## Prayer

God of the cross and the resurrection, allow us to keep our eyes on both, especially in the wake of our grief. Amen.

**R. P. Fugarino** is the Senior Minister at Park Hill Christian Church, Disciples of Christ, in Kansas City, Missouri.

# The God Who Listens

## Sharon A. Buttry

> *But I trust in you, O LORD;*
> *I say, "You are my God."*
> *My times are in your hand;*
> *deliver me from the hand of my enemies and*
> *persecutors. . . .*
> *I had said in my alarm,*
> *"I am driven far from your sight."*
> *But you heard my supplications*
> *when I cried out to you for help.* (Psalm 31:14-15, 22)

For me, the journey to motherhood was like walking down a long, lonely road with no true friend to hear my heart full of shame and pain. All my friends were having babies. Our fellowship group made quilts for each new arrival. I sewed each of my quilt square offerings with tears. I assumed God was blessing those women but not me. I did not even want to show up for worship or fellowship meetings with my sisters in Christ. My husband seemed fine—so much more secure in himself and not preoccupied with the emotional pain of infertility, at least not in the ways that I was.

My journey was seven years long. During that time I prayed, but it often seemed like my prayers were empty and hollow. I tried to take care of myself. I went to therapy, worked at my job at the Senior Center in Boston, and fulfilled my role as a pastor's wife. I had a public life that required me to present myself as a mature and joyful Christian, but inside I felt like a failure and so ashamed to be childless.

As time passed, I came to understand that I had choices to make in a situation that was not of my choosing. God's word became the centerpiece of how I began to interpret those choices. I found in Scripture many challenging scenarios that people did not choose and did not welcome. But inside each story, God was present and ready to listen to their hearts. Their characters were shaped on those long, lonely roads, with only God's ear to hear. The stories of Sarah, Moses, Tamar, Job, and Jeremiah all called to me. I made thousands of choices to hold on to the word, especially to God's promises to those who were barren, lonely, or grief-stricken. I began to realize that the people in the Bible were not super saints; they were ordinary people just like me, people whom God loves. A thousand times over, I chose to trust. I chose to have confidence that God was shaping me and my life, with or without children.

In many ways, God was giving birth to ME, so I could grow into motherhood. My way was to demand children for myself. God's answer to me was "you must become MY child first." I needed a lot of healing in my life, healing from childhood hurts and abuses. I needed to know God for myself, not through the church or fellowship meetings or my husband.

God took my hand on that lonely road and taught me how he listens. And I am a different person because of what I learned. Now I am able to claim that when I feel barren, when I feel lonely, when I feel wordless and tearful, when I feel a complete failure and a mess, when I am the most isolated and fearful, I am still God's child. I am never alone in my sorrow and grief because I am held in God's providence and cradled in God's love. The comfort I have received from God is a gift I choose to share every day as a mother, as a minister, and as a friend.

### Prayer

God, thank you for your faithful promise that you "draw near to those who draw near to you." Thank you for hearing the cries and meditations of my heart! Just like the sun is still high in the sky when the earth is covered with fog, sometimes I cannot feel your warmth and light. When grief blankets my heart, when disappointment clouds my view, remind me, God, that you are there listening to my prayer. Thank you for carrying me. Amen.

**Sharon A. Buttry** is currently Associate Director of Training and Education at the International Hope Center based in Hamtramck, Michigan. Rev. Buttry has extensive experience in urban ministry in the United States and has led workshops in social ministry and trauma awareness/recovery all over the world. She earned graduate degrees in ministry and social work in Philadelphia between 1992–1996 and was ordained in 1996 via the American Baptist Churches at Calvary Baptist Church of Norristown, Pennsylvania. She has been a leader in the Detroit area in interfaith relationships and serves as a voluntary police chaplain. She is a grant writer and administrator in community and police relations for Hamtramck. Rev. Buttry is married to Rev. Dr. Daniel Buttry, a Global Consultant for Peace and Justice, International Ministries, American Baptist Churches. Though they often travel for work, their home, Hopewell House, is a house they rescued from blight in Hamtramck, where they mentor ministry leaders. They are parents of three adult children who reside in Michigan and Texas. Rev. Buttry's interests include gardening, painting, and adventure camping.

# How Long?

## JENNIFER ANDREWS-WECKERLY

*How long, O LORD? Will you forget me forever? How long will you hide your face from me? How long must I bear pain in my soul, and have sorrow in my heart all day long? How long shall my enemy be exalted over me? Consider and answer me, O LORD my God!* (Psalm 13:1-3a)

"Aw, sh*t!" she exclaimed. I had just explained to one of my closest friends that I got my period, and we were not pregnant—yet again. This is why I always called her. She knew how brutal each month that passed could be. She knew the wave of emotions and the tensions that each month's failure brought. She never offered platitudes or acted like a cheerleader. She just let the profanities rip that were buried in my heart.

Beth was a blessing in my life during that time, more than she probably ever knew. She never assured me that things would work out, and she never filled the silence with encouragement. She asked insightful questions and named the things that I could not. Although she is not a priest, I often felt like our phone calls functioned as a confessional. She let me be angry with God, let me despair, and steadied me in the ambiguity. And I am sure that after our phone calls she lifted me in prayer.

Navigating friendships while trying to get pregnant was one of the most difficult components of the process. We did not tell many people in the first place because we were not sure how fertile we might be. We also did not want to face their faces of expectancy every month. But after several months of trying without success, while other friends were getting pregnant without even trying or at least after only a month or two of trying, my husband saw that I needed an outlet. He remembered that Beth and her husband had also struggled to get pregnant, and recommended that I reach out to her.

Beth was great because she understood both my faith life and my humanity. She understood the strain that trying to get pregnant put on a marriage. She understood the hopes and dreams that were constantly dashed. She understood that my prayer life and my theology were not always going to be in sync during this time.

By being able to handle all of my humanity, raw emotions, anger, disappointment, frustration, and sense of failure, Beth showed me God during that time. Her ability to take my pain and anger and still love me and see my love for God helped me see that God could do the same thing. God could handle my fickleness, my petulance, and my devastation. And just like Beth was ready by the phone at the drop of a hat, so was God. In her own way, Beth revealed God in the midst of all of it—without pedantically mentioning God.

Thinking back on that time, on the myriad times I cried out to God, "*How long, O LORD? How long?*" I now realize that God answered my prayers by giving me a beloved friend. God took the two of us—who had probably prayed this same psalm over and over again at different phases in our lives—and gave us each other. God did not answer me the way I wanted, but God did give me peace through my soul friend. I was not forgotten.

## *Prayer*

Generous God, we thank you for the blessing of holy companions for our journey. Help us to share our burdens with others, realizing that you often make yourself known to us through them. And though we might prefer our prayers to be answered in our own way, help us to remember that you are constantly seeking to answer our prayers as it may be best for us. Amen.

**Jennifer Andrews-Weckerly** joined the Episcopal Church of St. Margaret in December 2011 as the third rector in its forty-nine-year history. Prior to joining St. Margaret's, she completed a Bachelor of Arts in Political Science at Duke University in 1999. After a year of AmeriCorps service in North Carolina, Jennifer served as the Director of Volunteer Services at Habitat for Humanity of New Castle County, Delaware, for almost six years. Jennifer earned her Master in Divinity from Virginia Theological Seminary in May 2009. Upon graduation, she served as the Curate and Assistant Rector at Christ Church Christiana Hundred in Delaware for more than two years. Jennifer is married and has two daughters. She enjoys spending time with her family and friends, traveling, watching movies, and squeezing in a yoga or zumba class when she can. Her blog can be found at http://seekingandserving.wordpress.com.

# My Limits Confronted Me

## R. P. Fugarino

> *Bear one another's burdens, and in this way you will fulfill the law of Christ . . . . For all must carry their own loads.* (Galatians 6:2, 5)

The pregnancy sprung to life in our dark bedroom in Kansas City, Kansas. It bled to death a handful of weeks later in a tent on a sun-blasted dirt camping field in Juarez, Mexico. In the passionate intimacy of conceiving and in the horrible bloody intimacy of miscarrying, there were actions I performed and responsibilities I bore. There was a real power that was mine alone to wield, a load only I could carry.

But I also sensed that many things were always far beyond me and my abilities—an impotence of sorts. No, that's not quite right. A sense of impotence only struck me at the end, in the dying, when I knew there was nothing I could do to shield myself, my wife, or the pregnancy from the avalanche. I'll put it this way: through it all there was this sense of vulnerability, an exposure of self that was (and is)—irreducibly—both a blessing and a curse. I was confronted by my limits.

I knew this nakedness at the beginning of things when I thought about how much depended on the spastic, infinitesimal tails of my sperm. Did I have good swimmers? Or had I consumed too much diet soda as a child and somehow pickled and stunted them? And at the end there was this: when the doomed contractions were over—at least for the moment—and my wife rested from the lost battle, I stumbled from her bedside into the hospital waiting room. The dozen people who had traveled with us to Mexico to build a house rose to greet me.

They gathered around, laid hands on me, and prayed for the three of us. Their hands were not the heavy hands I remember feeling during my ordination. They were light, lifting hands seeking to take my shock and horror from me and toss them to heaven. Under them I was small and shattered, but also naked, unashamed, and blessed. Limited.

In Galatians 6, Paul has that weird, short span of four verses where he tells us that, especially in the midst of difficulty, we are both to bear one another's burdens and to carry our own loads.

Huh?

And yet this paradox is simply true to the way real life is lived by people who have limits to themselves and to their power. We follow Christ and seek to do it as well as we can, but we are also always gorgeous and fragile creatures who are limited and easily eclipsed. We have power, but things are often beyond our capabilities, and we often need to be carried.

I grieved that I was unable to make things work out the way we wanted. I was limited. However, my limits also made me a load that others could carry, and in this there was healing. In it, grace arrived for me as others raised me up in a hospital waiting room.

This is all still jumbled, even years later, but what I know is this: I didn't really feel the truth of Paul's words until my hands were soaked with my wife's blood and other, cleaner hands impressed upon me the love of the broken and risen One. In that moment, I knew I'd both carried my load and been carried by hands stronger than mine, and in that knowing, hope shone, subtly but surely.

Ten years later I still grieve the blood and death and seeing my limits in a hellish way I can't deny. Yet I still rejoice in being carried by Christ who works through the hands of his people. I am human and limited, and this is horrible, but it is also all right. Lord, have mercy.

## Prayer

God, whose Son came among us as and bears the limitations of our humanity, help us to see our own limitations not simply as curses, but also as opportunities for grace. Amen.

**R. P. Fugarino** is the Senior Minister at Park Hill Christian Church, Disciples of Christ, in Kansas City, Missouri.

# Movie People

## Brian Barrier

> *If then there is any encouragement in Christ, any consolation from love, any sharing in the Spirit, any compassion and sympathy, make my joy complete: be of the same mind, having the same love, being in full accord and of one mind.* (Philippians 2:1-4)

Every year I was in elementary school, there was a guy who would bring in his projector and home movies to show us in the cafeteria. Lots of rickety chairs were lined up, and we all paraded in on our best behavior because this was a special event and we would not want to miss it by being sent back to class.

All the movies were somewhat grainy, and the screen was quite small, but to us they were grand. We went to a small rural elementary school that ran from kindergarten to seventh grade. Many of us would never get to leave the confines of the state in our lifetime, much less travel to California to see giant redwood trees or drive in a car on the open road just to see where it took us. Heck, many of us didn't have a family that remotely resembled the one in the home movies. Yet here were these places in living color, rich food for our daydreams.

The people in the movies were a sign pointing to what we could have someday if we paid attention in class and worked hard enough. Someday, we too could be movie people that children would huddle together and stay quiet to see. Someday, God willing.

We all have our own movie people. Maybe they live on Facebook, sharing the warm glow of a birthday cake with their child who just turned five. Maybe they are in a supermarket, chatting to other parents as their children skip merrily down the aisles with miniature shopping carts. Maybe they are the parents hovering over a baby being pushed around a park in an awesomely decked-out stroller. Someday, God willing.

I remember when my wife Jenny and I prayed that prayer. We didn't really use those words. We just tried to do the right things. We paid attention in class. We worked hard. I had finally landed a job that paid a little more than barely enough to live on. My wife was going to graduate school. Jenny and I decided it may be the time to start a family. We made deals with God. In exchange for our hard work and devotion, God would surely grant us our dearest wish.

Jenny got pregnant. We decided to wait only a short while to tell everyone. My coworkers were planning a shower. Our friends were planning a shower. Jenny's belly was growing. The open road was in front of us, and we were driving just to see where it went. It felt like maybe, just maybe, we were going to be movie people too.

I was out of the state, training hospital workers on how to use disaster logistics software, when I got the call. Jenny had gone in for a routine ultrasound, and the technician could not find a heartbeat.

In elementary school, I remember when the home movies stopped. They usually wound down slowly after a parting shot with all of the movie people smiling and waving to the camera. There would be a profound silence. Then we would file out of the cafeteria back to our classrooms, but we were changed people. Sometimes it took a while for that to sink in.

It took a while for Jenny and I to get through the profound silence after our movie suddenly stopped. Folks didn't know what to say. Hallmark doesn't make a card for this situation.

I confess that I didn't know what to say or do either. The only times I had ever heard about miscarriage were in hushed tones with little context, as if one could somehow conjure it at will by speaking its name.

Then friends began to reach out to us and show us how things worked behind the scenes. We started hearing folks we thought of as movie people tell their own stories of loss, of frustration, of profound grief. They had tried to have children or had lost children. We never knew. Could this many folks have made the same deals with God?

The secret of the movie people paradigm is that we are the camera. We can choose where to look, what to focus on, and how the story will be told. I know that my experience with loss and grief has made me try to be a better participant in the lives of others, to better focus on them as real people. And this participation has taught me a lot about how our relationship with God is not transactional, not a talisman against loss to be conjured, but rather a sustained effort of engagement that allows us to express our deepest emotions while receiving the healing balm of encouragement.

Too easily we can get caught up in seeing folks just as they present themselves rather than getting to know them better. We need to tell others who have experienced the same loss, the same pain, the same grief, that they are not alone. Then perhaps we can begin to stand the movie people paradigm on its head. Someday, God willing.

## *Prayer*

Lord, please help us to see past the bright lights, listen past the memorized lines, and reach past the carefully hung backdrops of our communal stage to engage with the people around us. Thank you for the gifts of compassion and sympathy that remind us and help us to remind others that we are not alone and that all are loved.
In the name of Jesus Christ,
Amen.

Raised a Mennonite in rural Virginia, **Brian Barrier** now lives with his wife and two sons in Durham, North Carolina. He and his family attend Watts Street Baptist Church where he can often be found volunteering in one of the children's ministry classrooms. Brian is a computer programming specialist who uses his skills both professionally and in support of friends and neighbors who need computer support. Brian also enjoys gaming, poetry, and eclectic music.

# Everything Happens

## Holly Jarrell-Marcinelli

> *We know that all things work together for good for those who love God, who are called according to his purpose.* (Romans 8:28, NRSV)

> *And we know that in all things God works for the good of those who love him, who have been called according to his purpose.* (Romans 8:28, NIV)

My first IVF cycle capped off a long year and a half of trying to conceive, along with all the tests and procedures that go into establishing exactly why my partner and I would likely never conceive a child on our own. Imagine our relief to learn that the embryo transfer was a success, and on our first try we were pregnant! The call two days later that we were losing the pregnancy was crushing, and I watched the daydream images of our joyful pregnancy and children frolicking in the yard shatter around and within me. It was a feeling I will never forget.

    Three months later, we tried IVF again. Again, we were pregnant. This time the baby and I survived a relatively smooth forty-one-week pregnancy, and almost exactly one year after the date of our first failed IVF, I was holding our perfect daughter in my arms. When she was only a few days old, I said to my husband that if we hadn't had that miscarriage, then we wouldn't have had *her*. He wisely pointed out that if we hadn't had the miscarriage, then we would have had another baby, one whom we would have loved just as much, and we never once would have contemplated what it would be like to have a different baby. But I couldn't shake the weight of the importance of giving life not to just any child, but to *this* child. This child who will be different from any other person before her—who will grow to have her own personality, her own skills and talents, and hopefully her own God-loving heart to share with others. Like any parent, I often marvel that to know my daughter is not to be able to imagine a world without her. *Her.*

I write this while sitting on the couch in my doctor-prescribed two-day "couch potato" period, following our fourth ART cycle this year. The news this morning was good—an absolutely top-grade blastocyst is at this moment "hatching" and hopefully nestling into the perfect spot in my uterus to spend the next nine months. But this has been a year of one devastating disappointment after another. Certainly I didn't inject myself with hormones daily and go into three prior invasive procedures with the attitude that "well, this one isn't going to work, but we're doing it so that the time and circumstances can be laid in place to lead to our *fourth* procedure working." With our first cycle back in April, I fully expected it to work, and hoped that on this snowy December day I would be timing contractions and packing a hospital bag, not sitting on a couch praying for a microscopic grouping of cells to choose me for its home.

I told a friend recently that I'm not really an "everything happens for a reason" kind of person. I'm more of an "everything happens" person. I find it hard to swallow the idea that suffering is orchestrated into people's lives so that something else can happen. I think that suffering happens in everyone's life, and sometimes we can learn something from it, or salvage a good outcome, or at least a "better than nothing" outcome. Sometimes we can intervene to prevent suffering from falling into someone else's life. And when something good does come of something bad, we can be grateful and thank God for every blessing in our life. If no good is to be found, we keep trying, we keep going.

When I was in college, I wrote a paper on Romans 8:28, which I had learned growing up to read "All things work together for good . . . ." It is a translation that meshes well with the idea that God is an all-powerful puppeteer, masterminding everything that happens on earth to work together toward God's ultimate, good resolution. Since the creation of life, God has known how it all will end, having set in motion an impossible puzzle of fates and destinies all to come out right, or as God wills them, in the end.

The second translation above offers a different interpretation: "*In all things,* God works for good . . . ." A subtle but chasm-like difference. Has God known and planned all along that *this* time (or maybe next time, or maybe *no* time) is when I will get pregnant, because that fits into God's plan? Or is it that in the midst of the failings of my own body to fulfill the role to which I feel so strongly called, God will work to bring me comfort, or new opportunities, or a new understanding, or even a new calling? How comforting to know that God is in the jumble and ugliness of my disappointment and sorrow, mucking about and trying, with me, to shape things into a more acceptable, dare I hope "good," outcome.

So then, is it happening for a reason or not? While I may never be confident in the balance between God's power over the events of my life and my own responsibility to contribute to my destiny, I am forever grateful that whether God is the mastermind or the repairer, God is an active and present participant on this journey with me.

## Prayer

Oh God, only through your grace can I hope to have the faith to lay my will at your feet. Be present with me in this space where I fight for control and struggle to see the good. Open my eyes to your vision, and draw me to the place where my fears melt into trust and my pain becomes peace. Amen.

**Holly Jarrell-Marcinelli** attends Christ Church (Episcopal) in Andover, Massachusetts, where she serves as a verger, eucharistic minister, and a member of the Altar Guild. Holly is a licensed social worker, specializing in geriatric social work.

# From Chaos to Stillness

## Joy M. Freeman

> *God is our refuge and strength, a very present help in trouble. Therefore we will not fear, though the earth should change, though the mountains shake in the heart of the sea . . . .* (Psalm 46:1-2, NRSV)

The phone rang, and I saw it was the doctor's office. My heart jumped into my throat as panic began to pull at the edge of my being. I answered the phone, and my worst fears were realized: something was wrong with our baby, and a same-day appointment had already been made for us with the neonatologist. Panic now fully engulfed me, and what was a normal day turned to chaos. I wanted to pretend this was not happening; I hoped that if I ignored it, the reality of the situation would disappear. However, the professional chaplain in me prevailed. I had to face this. It was time to dive deeper into the chaos.

My husband and I went to the doctor, my heart pounding and crying out, "Please let them be wrong." We listened to the doctor's words: "Your baby has unsurvivable congenital anomalies." We saw the reality of these words on the big screen of the level 2 ultrasound, and the ground fell out from under me. I was thrust into a swirling chaos of thoughts and feelings. I could no longer tell where I began and ended and where the chaos began and ended. And so, when the doctor said that we needed to decide what we wanted to do, I did not think the chaos could go any deeper. Yet it did.

For the days to come, the questions pounded loudly in my head. *Why us, God? What did I do wrong? It had to have been my fault. I feel so broken. Why did this happen? How did this happen? Where in the world is God in all of this?* The questions swirled furiously; there were no good answers, and this was the hardest for me. As a chaplain, I am used to providing words of calm and peace. All I could hear was a deafening, scary, and painful silence.

Sometimes I was tempted to ask, "Was it something I did?" and "Why did God cause this to happen?" It was not something I did, and God did not cause it to happen. Yet the chaos makes us hear and believe many things that are neither helpful nor true. Our lives are so busy and so filled with noise that it is often impossible to accept the necessity of silence as something that can lead us to stillness and to a place of healing.

It was something my mother said that broke through the silence and began ushering me to stillness, that began to pull me out of the chaos. She reminded me of something I know to be true, something that in other circumstances I have been able to say to others: the God of perfection and love, who creates us in God's image, did not cause baby Hope to have those deformities or to die. Inexplicable things happen because the world is not perfect.

I needed to hear these words. They affirmed that God is in the middle of my situation, crying with me and carrying me through the chaos to the stillness of God's presence. In the stillness, I began to find healing and hear God's voice saying, "Let me in, and create something good out of this."

Now, several years later, sometimes the questions come back, but I hold firm to the truth that the God of love did not cause this but instead is here, working in me and through me, shaping my pain into something that, even from where I stand, I can call "good." This truth gives me the strength to stay out of the chaos and remain in the stillness of God's good work. This truth gives me the strength to tell my story and accompany other parents through the chaos toward the stillness, a privilege that, itself, provides healing.

## *Prayer*

God of the chaos and the stillness, stay close beside these parents who are in the middle of the deafening chaos and silence. Help them to know that you are holding the gut-wrenching questions in your hands in order to allow space in their lives for your calm and still presence. Guide them to the beginning of the journey to wholeness. Amen.

**Joy M. Freeman** graduated from Central Baptist Theological Seminary in 2001 with her Master of Divinity. She is an Endorsed American Baptist Chaplain and board certified through the Association of Professional Chaplains. She serves as a Critical Care and Maternity Chaplain at North Kansas City Hospital in the Kansas City Metro Area. She is also a Veriditas Certified Labyrinth Facilitator.

# That Much Faith

## Bekah Hart

> *He said to them, "Because of your little faith. For truly I tell you, if you have faith the size of a mustard seed, you will say to this mountain, 'Move from here to there,' and it will move; and nothing will be impossible for you."* (Matthew 17:20)

In Matthew 17:20, Jesus tells his disciples that their inability to heal a boy with a seizure disorder is directly related to their lack of faith. His admonishment comes with an illustration that was probably a slap in the face. Jesus tells those he had lived with, prayed with, and taught that they only need the faith of a tiny mustard seed to do things that might ordinarily be impossible.

Surviving stillbirth seems impossible. I do it every day, and it still seems impossible. A living, breathing part of me was buried in a small white box in a clearing on a mountainside. How does one survive that?

I used to think that my older sister was super-human. After eight months of pregnancy and a grueling labor, she left the hospital with empty arms and went home to a crumbling marriage. "Regular people don't survive that," I thought. Then I did it. My marriage wasn't crumbling, but I, too, went home with empty, aching arms and a battered and broken heart. How do we do it?

When I was in labor, I repeatedly asked how women did this. How do we put our bodies through such pain and survive? How do some of us go through this, go home with no baby, grieve for a lifetime, and survive? My husband repeatedly assured me that I was surviving the agony of labor and that I would survive the eternal heartbreak of loss.

About a month after my son's funeral, my sister gave me a necklace. It had a heart engraved with his name, "Silas," and his birthday, and it had a cross with his birthstone in the center. She also told me that I was welcome to add to it the mustard-seed pendant that she had worn after her son's death. Though I knew that the pendant itself was not some kind of magic charm, it felt right and meaningful and comforting to wear something she had worn during a similar time.

After she gave it to me, she told me something that transformed the mustard seed as an illustration object for faith. She said she had stopped viewing it as the rebuke Jesus gave to the disciples to "have more faith." Instead, when her life was falling apart, she gathered up all of her confidence, looked at the mustard seed, and said, "That's tiny. Surely I have *that* much faith."

So I added it to the necklace and wore it daily. Whenever I thought that there was no way I was going to survive the hymn we sang at his funeral, the baby crying in the cereal aisle at Target, or my pregnancy with Silas's younger brother, I would reach up and touch the mustard seed. Then I'd plot the quickest way out, dig the wad of tissue from my bag, and lose it. Knowing I had the faith to make it didn't mean I was a rock; it meant that when I was out of tears and my cheeks were black with mascara, I'd have enough faith to make it to the next breakdown.

Survival is something that happens over and over again, not merely once or twice, and not always because of conscious decisions. You will survive. Like me, like my sister, like so many others who have lived the heartbreak of loss, you, friend, have "that much faith." And "that much faith" is the only way you learn to survive. Hour by hour. Day by day. Tear by tear.

My sister and I have faith. We have faith that our God grieves our sons, just as he grieved his own. We have faith that, though the world we live in now is fallen, God will work redemptively to bring about the world as God intended. Faith doesn't mean we're okay with, or understand, our children's deaths. It doesn't mean we think that their deaths are part of some greater plan. Instead, we've chosen to place our faith in a companion and comforter on this shared journey of anguishing grief.

## Prayer

God of comfort and peace, overwhelm us with your calming presence and give us the faith we need to face each new day. Amen.

> **Bekah Hart** is the mother of two beautiful redheaded boys—one she didn't get to keep and one she snuggles extra close. She is a former field personnel with the Cooperative Baptist Fellowship and currently works as a nanny. She lives in Rock Hill, South Carolina, with her husband, Blake, and younger son, Benji, where they are members of Oakland Baptist Church. She enjoys refinishing furniture, eating cookie dough, and making to-do lists.

# Barrenness and HOPE

## Pam Durso

> *Zechariah and Elizabeth were righteous before God, living blamelessly according to all the commandments and regulations of the Lord. But they had no children, because Elizabeth was barren, and both were getting on in years.* (Luke 1:6-7)

Barrenness is such a lonely word. Hearing it and reading it always leaves me feeling alone and a little lost.

In the first chapter of Luke's Gospel, the writer tells us that Zechariah and Elizabeth lived with barrenness for many, many years (Luke 1:5-23, 57-80). They not only suffered pain over having no children but also experienced humiliation, disgrace, and embarrassment. In their day, children were signs of God's favor—demonstrations of God's blessing. Having no children meant that God was withholding blessings from this devoutly religious couple.

Most likely, Elizabeth was the one who bore the burden for their infertility. In the first century, the wife was most often held responsible for a couple's barrenness, and thus Elizabeth took on that blame. She was the one who brought disgrace to herself and to her husband. But Zechariah suffered right along with her. He too knew pain, and he too was heartbroken. These two sad, hurting people, a married couple longing for a miracle, wished desperately for a child. But they were too old, much too old to be having a baby.

This is not a happy story—and in fact, it seems to be a hopeless one. Is there any good news, any hope for this elderly married couple named Zechariah and Elizabeth? We all know how this story ends. We know about the miracle. We know that Elizabeth will soon be pregnant. We know that she births a son that they will name John.

In the end, this truly is a story of hope, but I would like to go out on a limb and say that the HOPE I find in this text is not Elizabeth's pregnancy or the birth of John the Baptist. Elizabeth's miraculous conception at a very old age and the safe delivery of a tiny baby boy is not what makes this passage a story of HOPE for me.

Instead, HOPE is found in unexpected places. Hope does not come suddenly at the end of the story, and hope is not just wishful thinking about the future. Instead, hope is written between the lines of this text. Hope is hidden in curious parts of this passage. Hope is found in the everyday routines of this couple. Hope shows up while Zechariah is fulfilling his priestly duties, serving every day at his job in the temple. Hope is found in the words of promise spoken by the angel to a doubting Zechariah. Hope grows stronger in the sacredness of Zechariah's silence. Hope is seen in unexpected places.

I must confess, however, that I have often rushed through the first twenty-two verses of this chapter of Luke, hurrying toward verse 57—rushing to read "she gave birth to a son." Those words are the highlight for me, the good part of the story, the happy ending.

During my years of living with infertility, I needed stories with happy endings. I needed HOPE that a baby would come to us. I needed somehow to believe that God would do a miracle. I needed my own happy ending!

Twenty years later, I still like happy endings. I like stories that conclude with miracles, and my personal story has had a few miracles along the way. In 1994 and again in 1997, through the miracle of adoption, my husband and I became parents. We received good news that babies would indeed come to us.

But despite my continuing desire for happy endings, as I have aged I have become much less willing to skip the first part of Luke 1. Those first verses have become more important, more meaningful, more helpful to me than the latter verses, for I have learned that you can't skip to the end when it comes to life. You can't avoid the hardness or pain of living. You can't avoid the challenging times. You have to deal with the struggle.

I have also learned that sometimes a good ending isn't the ending at all but only a new beginning. Our adoption of Michael and Alex began a whole new phase of our lives—we became parents and have experienced all the joys and frustrations and insanity and hardships that go with parenting.

And I have also learned that sometimes—well, many times—there is not a happy ending. Some stories don't end well. Sometimes there isn't a miracle.

So what do we do? How do we live with HOPE in the midst of pain, heartbreak, doubt, uncertainty, questions? We can find hope as we live faithfully day by day. We can find hope in the midst of sincere doubts. We can find hope even on those days when our faith is in short supply, and we can find hope in the quiet times, in times of silence.

Our hope is not just wishful thinking about the future or dreams of what can be. Our hope grows out of reliance on God. Our hope comes from our connection with God's purposes and our desire for God's presence. Our hope is in the God who holds our future, but our hope is also in our God who is with us now, our God who gives us the strength to deal with the chaos of life, with the hurts and suffering that we all encounter.

Our HOPE is in God.

## Prayer

God of HOPE, may we sense your presence and your love in our times of hopelessness. And on those days when we feel most alone and disconnected, give us the strength and courage to hold on to hope. Amen.

> **Pam Durso** is the executive director of Baptist Women in Ministry, an independent Baptist organization that supports and advocates for Baptist women ministers. She loves walking alongside and encouraging women called by God to ministry. Pam also enjoys researching, writing, and teaching in the area of Baptist history. She teaches Baptist history as an adjunct professor at McAfee School of Theology. She and her husband, Keith, live in Lawrenceville, Georgia, with their son, Michael, and daughter, Alex.

# Life under Heaven Lives with What Is

## Mary McMillan Terry

> *The heavens are telling the glory of God;*
> *and the firmament proclaims his handiwork.*
> *Day to day pours forth speech,*
> *and night to night declares knowledge.*
> *There is no speech, nor are there words;*
> *their voice is not heard;*
> *yet their voice goes out through all the earth,*
> *and their words to the end of the world.*
> *In the heavens he has set a tent for the sun,*
> *which comes out like a bridegroom from his wedding canopy,*
> *and like a strong man runs its course with joy.*
> *Its rising is from the end of the heavens,*
> *and its circuit to the end of them;*
> *and nothing is hid from its heat.* (Psalm 19:1-6)

The heavens that September day were full of sun that shone down on my dark head. There were no words, though, as the psalm says, and that was good because I wasn't listening. My head was full with news of what was lost.

My husband and I had spent the previous four months planning with a doctor in a not-so-nearby city a cycle of in-vitro fertilization. After three years of failed attempts at conception, including unsuccessful medical interventions, we had launched headlong that previous spring into IVF, a decision weighty in cost and time. One that included spending twenty thousand dollars, injecting medications daily (or sometimes more) for six weeks, and driving hundreds of miles for procedures and monitoring.

As I walked into our condo complex that September day, I felt the pavement at my feet. The process of IVF had felt productive, like taking concrete steps toward fulfilling a shared desire. The precise protocols, the prescriptions and indications: this was work, but with it grew the hope that joy instead of infertility might mark our path. But now the embryo—implanted alive days before—was dead, and so were we, in a way. I wandered, untethered and unaware of any productive next step.

It was hard to listen, in the wake of this loss, to anything: a physician's advice, friends' condolences, even prayers. So many questions, regrets, and attempts to make sense of the experience circled in my head. I found, though, that memorization—the repetitive and uneventful nature of it—helped silence roving thoughts and settle my soul. So during walks I took around our condo complex that month, I repeated Psalm 19.

The psalm's orientation is vertical, and thus its words reminded me, prone at the time to allowing my eyes to fall, to look up. The reorienting lent me badly needed perspective. Even breathing is more difficult when grief shrinks one's world to the patch of ground beneath one's feet.

At the same time, the psalm's "no" and "nor" lent lexical location for me to hang my negative energy. There had been no words to sustain the life of our child. As I walked with this psalm, I felt its words expand, as if breathing, to contain, to hold within it my life, which now included our child's death.

My husband walked with me at times. We both needed, it seemed, the space the heavens gave to grieve. And though I won't say I witnessed the glory of God on those walks, I did hear my husband's tenor voice reminding me, and us, that Christ, the suffering servant, surely was suffering with us.

And I did believe, in perhaps the most elementary way—by sight. I believed in the heavens, their billowing blue above my head. Their clouds that filtered the roving and restless sun. Surely nothing is hidden from its heat, a fact I found oppressive and reassuring.

For the sun of Psalm 19 is Christ, the wandering Jew, who sees what we see but refuses, simultaneously, to stay a distant god. Instead, Christ comes to us a bridegroom, a strong man.

The day-to-day testified to in the psalm paced my step-by-step movement through days and weeks of grief. Survival depends, depended for me, on simple steps and even shallow breaths.

It is in such unexceptional movement, in walking out of a reality we didn't want but find ourselves experiencing, that we keep on living.

And indeed, our unexceptional movement becomes exceptional. For if the sun in this psalm is Christ, it is also us, believers in whom Christ lives. And his life in us is the hope of glory (Col 1:27). Hope that we, strong women and men of God, will walk and sometimes run our course, our actual one, not the one we hoped for but the one that is. That is God's glory. That we walk, day to day, night to night, knowing that in our walking, knowledge is revealed to us and to others.

## Prayer

God who created all that is firm and of this earth, and all that is beyond in the glorious heavens, form us in our grief. Help us to stay the course, the course that is our course, the course unfolding before us in all its joy and pain and mystery. Help us to live with what is. Amen.

**Mary McMillan Terry** teaches composition and American literature at Pellissippi State Community College in Knoxville, Tennessee, where she lives with her husband and two sons. Her writing has been published or is forthcoming in *Switched-On Gutenberg: A Global Poetry Journal*, *In Touch Magazine*, *Appalachian Heritage*, *Ebola* chapbook (published by West Chester University), *Autumn Magic* (the 2014 Durham Editing and E-books Autumn Anthology), *The Continuum Encyclopedia of Young Adult Literature*,

*The Zinnia Tales* (a collection of short stories published by Mountain Girl Press), and *The Salt and Light Handbook: A Guide to Loving Knoxville*. She holds a master's degree in literature from the University of Tennessee and a BA in English from UNC-Chapel Hill.

# Shambles

## WILLIAM JOSEPH (B. J.) HUTTO

*Set your minds on things that are above, not on things that are on earth, for you have died, and your life is hidden with Christ in God. When Christ who is your life is revealed, then you also will be revealed with him in glory.* (Colossians 3:2-3)

No one tells you when you're young that you'll feel ridiculous during some of the most important moments of your life. If you were raised on American pop culture like I was, you come to expect that those moments on which life pivots will contain a certain gravitas: John Cusack, feet firmly planted in the soil, hoisting a boom box toward his love; Tom Cruise valiantly tossing Goose's dog tags into the sea; Ferris Bueller's friend, Cameron, finally deciding to be brave enough to confront his father. You come to expect a scene worthy of the moment, worthy of remembering.

And so, on the day that I retrieved my unborn daughter's ashes from the funeral home all the way down on 14th Street, it was a shock to realize that I could feel so foolish as I sat on the L train. Foolish because the box—all cheap, shiny white plastic and severe right angles—refused to fit inside the bag that I had brought to hide it. Foolish because as I sat there cradling in my lap this bulging, unclosed bag, these few tiny ashes, a woman—clearly within days of her due date—sat across from me in morbid juxtaposition.

And so, on the day that my wife and I drove to the Atlantic Ocean to return the dust of our daughter's bones to the dust of the earth, it was a shock that an occasion so solemn could be so awkward. The stiff breeze blowing in off the water made scattering Mary's ashes with any dignity impossible, so I was compelled to wade in and return her not via wind but via wave: wave upon wave, waiting for the tide to finally rinse clean the disposable plastic baggy in my hands (tied, of course, with a predictably uncooperative wire tie). And then what does one do afterward with the baggy, with the box, with the tie? Sometimes life really is a shambles.

In those uncomfortable moments and in returning to those uncomfortable moments, it is crucial that we remind ourselves that our lives are not lived out before a crowd, bared for the world on some big screen, but are instead hidden—"encrypted," almost, in the original Greek—in the life of Christ: the child who had to flee from Herod to postpone death; the man who refused to flee from Pilate, thereby submitting to death; the Messiah, nail-pierced and scourged, whose resurrection swore that he, and not death and his minions, will have the final word. We belong to him, as do our children. Our lives and their lives are hidden in his. Our lives' logic, their meaning, their *telos* are hidden in his, not in some sense of drama or solemnity. And this means that all of our lives are, along with his, actually yet to be revealed, revealed to one another, to the world, and even to ourselves. There is life yet. Scars may remain. Suffering will not. Tears will not. This is the hope that we've been given, for if Christ is not raised from the dead, then we above all people are to be most pitied (1 Cor 15:19), but if he is—and he is—then we know that none of our stories, nor any of theirs, will be fully written until that final day.

## Prayer

Loving God, as we and our families trudge through the broken places of your creation, keep us ever mindful of the glorious resurrection of your broken Son, Jesus Christ, and of our promised share in his coming kingdom. Just as we live only in his life, we pray this prayer in his name. Amen.

**William Joseph (B. J.) Hutto** is an ordained Baptist minister and is currently completing his PhD in theological ethics, at-distance, at the University of Aberdeen (Scotland).

# Index

Abraham 67–69, 72, 84

Adoption 84, 144

Advent 26, 58, 79–80

Anger ix, 20, 26, 29–31, 33–34, 40, 44, 53–54, 57, 62–63, 65–66, 68–69, 93, 100, 120

Ashes 43, 62, 151

Baby xi, 6, 9–10, 13–15, 19, 25–26, 29–30, 33, 39–40, 44, 49–50, 53, 57, 67–68, 71, 77, 79, 83–84, 99–100, 104, 107–108, 127, 131, 135–36, 139–40, 143–44

Bed rest xii

Birth (see also Live birth) x, 6, 15, 34, 50, 53, 62, 68, 77, 79, 107–109, 116, 143–44

Blood 87, 95, 124

Body 16, 20, 29–30, 36, 39, 53–54, 61–62, 68, 87–88, 91, 99–100, 107, 133

Chaplain 10–11, 17, 34, 39–40, 45, 47–49, 51, 62–63, 83, 86, 117, 135, 137

Child(ren) i, ix, v, vii, xii, xiii, 5–7, 9–11, 13, 14–16, 19–20, 21, 24, 25, 27, 29, 33, 39–40, 43, 47, 49, 54, 57–58, 61, 65, 66–68, 77, 79, 83–85, 86, 87, 88–89, 91, 92, 95–97, 99, 100, 103, 104, 108, 111–12, 116–17, 123, 127–29, 131, 140, 143, 148, 152

Conceive(d) 68, 83–84, 104, 109, 131

Conception 84, 91, 111, 144, 147

Congregation(s) 17, 84, 111

Cried xi, 15, 19–20, 43, 62, 84, 99–100, 107, 115, 120

Cry 20, 23–24, 43–44, 47, 50, 53–54, 69, 100

Crying ix, 3, 7, 30, 50, 68, 92, 135–36, 140

Dark(est) x, xii, 1, 7, 35, 49, 62, 66, 68–69, 71–73, 77, 83, 87, 100, 103, 108, 123, 147

Darkness i–ii, vii–viii, x, xii, 1–2, 6, 8, 10, 14, 16, 20, 24, 26, 30, 34, 36, 40, 44, 48, 50, 54, 58, 62, 65–66, 68, 71–72, 75, 77–78, 80, 84–86, 88, 92, 96, 100, 104, 108, 112, 116, 120, 124, 128, 132, 136, 140, 144, 148, 150, 152

Death i–ii, xi, 19, 23–24, 26–27, 43–44, 47, 71–72, 104, 108, 112, 123–24, 140, 148, 152

Delivery room 62

Depressed 72

Depression 6, 10

Died/Dying 9–11, 19–20, 25, 77, 87, 88, 108, 112, 123, 151

Doctor 9, 13–14, 19–20, 39, 62, 84, 95, 104, 132, 135, 147

Elizabeth 143

Empty 6, 24, 36, 62, 67, 72, 80, 115, 139

Expecting x–xi, 13, 19, 79–81

Faith i, x–xii, 2, 5, 7, 20, 44, 58, 61–63, 66, 71–72, 83–85, 96, 99–100, 120, 133, 139–41, 145

Family(ies) xii, 1, 6, 8, 15–16, 19–20, 25, 27, 33, 35, 47, 59, 71, 78–79, 84, 86, 91–93, 96, 104, 107–108, 121, 127–29, 152

Father 14, 17, 39, 99, 111–12, 151

Forget(ting) xi, 5, 44, 63, 78, 87–89, 104, 107, 119, 131

Funeral, 139–40, 151

Grief i, v, vii, ix–x, xii, 1–2, 7, 9–11, 14–17, 20, 23–27, 29–30, 33–36, 39–40, 43, 47–50, 53–54, 62, 68, 77–78, 83–85, 88–89, 91–92, 96, 100, 105, 107, 112–13, 116, 128–29, 140, 148–49

Grieve ix, 9–11, 15, 24, 26–27, 48, 61, 78, 95, 124, 139, 148

Hannah 5–7

Hannah Ministry, xiii, 8, 31, 78

Help(s) i, x, 9–11, 24, 35, 36, 39–40, 43–44, 50, 53–54, 58, 63, 66, 72, 80, 85, 91–93, 96, 99–100, 115, 120, 124, 129, 135–36, 149

Helpless 9, 35, 79, 87

Home xii, 13, 24–25, 62, 85, 101, 117, 127–28, 132, 139, 151

Hope i, vii, x, xii, 2, 7–8, 13–17, 19–20, 23–24, 27, 29–30, 37, 47, 49–50, 63, 72, 77, 79–81, 83–85, 92, 96, 99–100, 103, 108, 116, 124, 133, 136, 143–45, 148–49, 152

Hospital 1, 15, 24–25, 40, 43–44, 47, 49, 51, 65, 77, 83, 86, 123–24, 128, 132, 137, 139

Husband xiii, 5–7, 10–11, 14, 19, 29–30, 36, 40, 61–63, 67–69, 79, 83–84, 89, 91, 96–97, 100, 104, 115–16, 119, 131, 135, 139, 141, 143–45, 147–49

In-vitro fertilization 84, 147

Infertility i–ii, xi–xiii, 1–2, 5–7, 53, 65–68, 77, 79–80, 84, 91, 93, 107–109, 115, 143–44, 148

IVF 79–80, 109, 131, 147–48

Jealousy 49–50, 93

Journey 6, 15, 17, 20, 37, 48, 50, 58, 65–66, 80, 83–85, 89, 91–93, 115, 120, 133, 136, 140

Live birth, 53

Loss i–ii, v, xi–xiii, 1–2, 9–11, 14, 16, 26–27, 29, 35–37, 40–41, 43, 47–48, 53, 68, 71, 77, 83–84, 88–89, 92, 95–96, 103, 112, 128–29, 139–40, 148

Lost 8, 10, 16, 20, 24, 26, 29–30, 33, 37, 62, 65, 71, 77, 79, 87–89, 95, 100, 104, 123, 128, 143, 147

Marriage 36–37, 68, 103–104, 107, 120, 139

# INDEX

Mary 57–58

Miscarriage i–ii, xi–xii, 1–2, 9–10, 16, 34–37, 53, 65, 71, 84, 87, 89, 104, 111, 128, 131

Miscarrier 53

Mother 9, 13–14, 33, 39–40, 49, 53, 68, 83–84, 92, 112, 116, 136, 141

Motherhood i–ii, 7, 61, 83, 91, 115–16

Obstetrician xi, 29, 91

Parent(s) 14, 20, 24–25, 33, 41, 49–50, 67, 83, 100, 117, 127, 131, 136, 144

Partner ix, 36, 39, 57, 59, 131

Peace 15–16, 34, 37, 54, 62, 100, 117, 120, 133, 135, 141

Pregnancy(ies) xi–xiii, 1, 10, 13, 16, 19, 24, 28, 33–34, 36, 39, 41, 53–54, 58, 61, 71, 77, 81–84, 88, 92, 101, 103, 107, 111, 123, 131, 139–40, 144

Pregnant xii, 9, 13–14, 19, 53, 57–58, 68, 79–80, 91, 93, 99, 107, 119–20, 128, 131, 133, 143

Rage i, 1–2, 7–8, 30, 78

Sarah 67–69, 85, 116

Sibling(s) 15, 25–26, 80

Silence i, ix, xi, 10, 35, 37, 39–40, 63, 80, 93, 119, 128, 135–36, 144–45, 148

Silent 37, 44, 66, 96

Soul xi, 5–6, 15–17, 29–30, 43, 69, 72, 88, 119–20, 148

Stillbirth ii, 111, 139

Suffer(ing) v, x, 9, 36–37, 62, 99, 104, 107–109, 132, 145, 148, 152

Surgery(ies) 13, 15, 107

Tears 8, 10, 15, 19, 23–24, 26, 35, 39, 47, 50, 67, 84, 89, 92, 100, 107, 115, 140, 152

Twins 19, 92

Ultrasound xii, 19, 29, 61, 128, 135

Wait xii, 6, 15, 17, 49, 79–81, 93, 128

Waiting xi–xii, 19, 25, 50, 65, 80, 92–93, 95, 123–24, 151

Waiting room xi, 65, 123–24

Wife v, xi, 6, 16, 24, 35–37, 39, 65, 67, 107, 109, 111, 115, 123–24, 128–29, 143, 151

Womb(s) 5, 36, 57, 65, 68, 85, 87, 88, 95–96

Zechariah 143–44

*Other available titles from*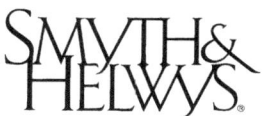

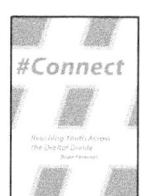

### #Connect
Reaching Youth Across the Digital Divide
*Brian Foreman*

Reaching our youth across the digital divide is a struggle for parents, ministers, and other adults who work with Generation Z—today's teenagers. #*Connect* leads readers into the technological landscape, encourages conversations with teenagers, and reminds us all to be the presence of Christ in every facet of our lives.   978-1-57312-693-9  120 pages/pb  **$13.00**

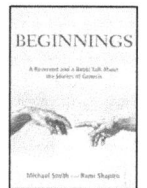

### Beginnings
A Reverend and a Rabbi Talk About the Stories of Genesis
*Michael Smith and Rami Shapiro*

Editor Aaron Herschel Shapiro describes storytelling as an "infinite game" because stories "must be retold—not just repeated, but reinvented, reimagined, and reexperienced" to remain vital in the world. Mike and Rami continue their conversations from the *Mount and Mountain* books, exploring the places where their traditions intersect and diverge, listening to each other as they respond to the stories of creation, of Adam and Eve, Cain and Abel, Noah, Jacob, and Joseph.   978-1-57312-772-1  202 pages/pb  **$18.00**

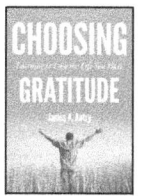

### Choosing Gratitude
Learning to Love the Life You Have
*James A. Autry*

Autry reminds us that gratitude is a choice, a spiritual—not social—process. He suggests that if we cultivate gratitude as a way of being, we may not change the world and its ills, but we can change our response to the world. If we fill our lives with moments of gratitude, we will indeed love the life we have.   978-1-57312-614-4  144 pages/pb  **$15.00**

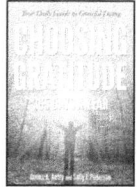

### Choosing Gratitude 365 Days a Year
Your Daily Guide to Grateful Living
*James A. Autry and Sally J. Pederson*

Filled with quotes, poems, and the inspired voices of both Pederson and Autry, in a society consumed by fears of not having "enough"—money, possessions, security, and so on—this book suggests that if we cultivate gratitude as a way of being, we may not change the world and its ills, but we can change our response to the world.   978-1-57312-689-2  210 pages/pb  **$18.00**

To order call **1-800-747-3016** or visit **www.helwys.com**

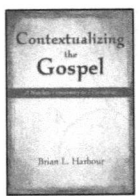
### Contextualizing the Gospel
#### A Homiletic Commentary on 1 Corinthians
*Brian L. Harbour*

Harbour examines every part of Paul's letter, providing a rich resource for those who want to struggle with the difficult texts as well as the simple texts, who want to know how God's word—all of it—intersects with their lives today.  978-1-57312-589-5  240 pages/pb  **$19.00**

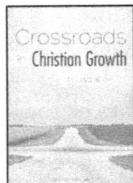
### Crossroads in Christian Growth
*W. Loyd Allen*

Authentic Christian life presents spiritual crises and we struggle to find a hero walking with God at a crossroads. With wisdom and sincerity, W. Loyd Allen presents Jesus as our example and these crises as stages in the journey of growth we each take toward maturity in Christ.  978-1-57312-753-0  164 pages/pb  **$15.00**

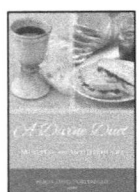
### A Divine Duet
#### Ministry and Motherhood
*Alicia Davis Porterfield, ed.*

Each essay in this inspiring collection is as different as the mother-minister who wrote it, from theologians to chaplains, inner-city ministers to rural-poverty ministers, youth pastors to preachers, mothers who have adopted, birthed, and done both.  978-1-57312-676-2  146 pages/pb  **$16.00**

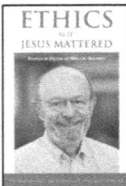
### Ethics as if Jesus Mattered
#### Essays in Honor of Glen H. Stassen
*Rick Axtell, Michelle Tooley, Michael L. Westmoreland-White, eds.*

*Ethics as if Jesus Mattered* will introduce Stassen's work to a new generation, advance dialogue and debate in Christian ethics, and inspire more faithful discipleship just as it honors one whom the contributors consider a mentor.  978-1-57312-695-3  234 pages/pb  **$18.00**

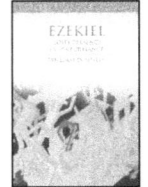
### Ezekiel (Smyth & Helwys Annual Bible Study series)
#### God's Presence in Performance
*William D. Shiell*

Through a four-session Bible study for individuals and groups, Shiell interprets the book of Ezekiel as a four-act drama to be told to adult, children, and youth groups living out their faith in a strange, new place. The book encourages congregations to listen to God's call, accept where God has planted them, surrender the shame of their past, receive a new heart from God, and allow God to breathe new life into them.

*Teaching Guide* 978-1-57312-755-4  192 pages/pb  **$14.00**
*Study Guide* 978-1-57312-756-1  126 pages/pb  **$6.00**

**To order call 1-800-747-3016 or visit www.helwys.com**

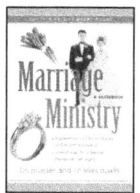
### Marriage Ministry: A Guidebook
*Bo Prosser and Charles Qualls*

This book is equally helpful for ministers, for nearly/newlywed couples, and for thousands of couples across our land looking for fresh air in their marriages.  1-57312-432-X  150 pages/pb  **$16.00**

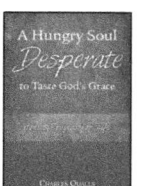
### A Hungry Soul Desperate to Taste God's Grace
### Honest Prayers for Life
*Charles Qualls*

Part of how we *see* God is determined by how we *listen* to God. There is so much noise and movement in the world that competes with images of God. This noise would drown out God's beckoning voice and distract us. Charles Qualls's newest book offers readers prayers for that journey toward the meaning and mystery of God.  978-1-57312-648-9  152 pages/pb  **$14.00**

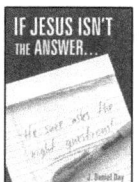
### If Jesus Isn't the Answer . . . He Sure Asks the Right Questions!
*J. Daniel Day*

Taking eleven of Jesus' questions as its core, Day invites readers into their own conversation with Jesus. Equal parts testimony, theological instruction, pastoral counseling, and autobiography, the book is ultimately an invitation to honest Christian discipleship.

978-1-57312-797-4  148 pages/pb  **$16.00**

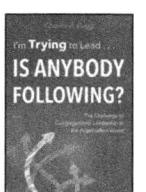
### I'm Trying to Lead . . . Is Anybody Following?
### The Challenge of Congregational Leadership in the Postmodern World
*Charles B. Bugg*

Bugg provides us with a view of leadership that has theological integrity, honors the diversity of church members, and reinforces the brave hearts of church leaders who offer vision and take risks in the service of Christ and the church.  978-1-57312-731-8  136 pages/pb  **$13.00**

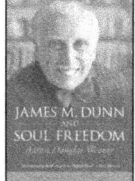
### James M. Dunn and Soul Freedom
*Aaron Douglas Weaver*

James Milton Dunn, over the last fifty years, has been the most aggressive Baptist proponent for religious liberty in the United States. Soul freedom—voluntary, uncoerced faith and an unfettered individual conscience before God—is the basis of his understanding of church-state separation and the historic Baptist basis of religious liberty.  978-1-57312-590-1  224 pages/pb  **$18.00**

**To order call 1-800-747-3016 or visit www.helwys.com**

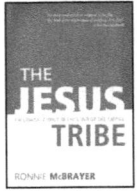
### The Jesus Tribe
#### Following Christ in the Land of the Empire
*Ronnie McBrayer*

The Jesus Tribe fleshes out the implications, possibilities, contradictions, and complexities of what it means to live within the Jesus Tribe and in the shadow of the American Empire.

978-1-57312-592-5  208 pages/pb  **$17.00**

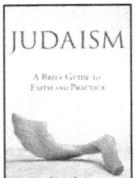
### Judaism
#### A Brief Guide to Faith and Practice
*Sharon Pace*

Sharon Pace's newest book is a sensitive and comprehensive introduction to Judaism. What is it like to be born into the Jewish community? How does belief in the One God and a universal morality shape the way in which Jews see the world? How does one find meaning in life and the courage to endure suffering? How does one mark joy and forge community ties?

978-1-57312-644-1  144 pages/pb  **$16.00**

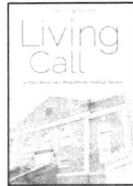
### Living Call
#### An Old Church and a Young Minister Find Life Together
*Tony Lankford*

This light look at church and ministry highlights the dire need for fidelity to the vocation of church leadership. It also illustrates Lankford's conviction that the historic, local congregation has a beautiful, vibrant, and hopeful future.

978-1-57312-702-8  112 pages/pb  **$12.00**

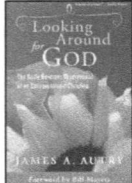
### Looking Around for God
#### The Strangely Reverent Observations of an Unconventional Christian
*James A. Autry*

*Looking Around for God*, Autry's tenth book, is in many ways his most personal. In it he considers his unique life of faith and belief in God. Autry is a former Fortune 500 executive, author, poet, and consultant whose work has had a significant influence on leadership thinking.

978-157312-484-3  144 pages/pb  **$16.00**

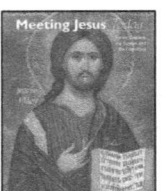
### Meeting Jesus Today
#### For the Cautious, the Curious, and the Committed
*Jeanie Miley*

*Meeting Jesus Today*, ideal for both individual study and small groups, is intended to be used as a workbook. It is designed to move readers from studying the Scriptures and ideas within the chapters to recording their journey with the Living Christ.

978-1-57312-677-9  320 pages/pb  **$19.00**

---

**To order call 1-800-747-3016 or visit www.helwys.com**

### The Ministry Life
#### 101 Tips for Ministers' Spouses
*John and Anne Killinger*

While no pastor does his or her work alone, roles for a spouse or partner are much more flexible and fluid in the twenty-first century than they once were. Spouses who want to support their minister-mates' vocation may wonder where to begin. The Killingers' suggestions are notable for their range of interests; whatever your talents may be, the Killingers have identified a way to put those gifts to work in tasks both large and small.

978-1-57312-769-1  252 pages/pb  **$19.00**

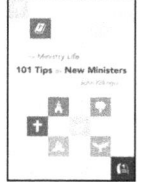
### The Ministry Life
#### 101 Tips for New Ministers
*John Killinger*

Sharing years of wisdom from more than fifty years in ministry and teaching, The Ministry Life: 101 Tips for New Ministers by John Killinger is filled with practical advice and wisdom for a minister's day-to-day tasks as well as advice on intellectual and spiritual habits to keep ministers of any age healthy and fulfilled.

978-1-57312-662-5  244 pages/pb  **$19.00**

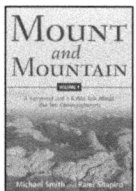
### Mount and Mountain
#### Vol. 1: A Reverend and a Rabbi Talk About the Ten Commandments
*Rami Shapiro and Michael Smith*

Mount and Mountain represents the first half of an interfaith dialogue—a dialogue that neither preaches nor placates but challenges its participants to work both singly and together in the task of reinterpreting sacred texts. Mike and Rami discuss the nature of divinity, the power of faith, the beauty of myth and story, the necessity of doubt, the achievements, failings, and future of religion, and, above all, the struggle to live ethically and in harmony with the way of God.

978-1-57312-612-0  144 pages/pb  **$15.00**

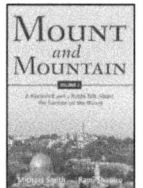
### Mount and Mountain
#### Vol. 2: A Reverend and a Rabbi Talk About the Sermon on the Mount
*Rami Shapiro and Michael Smith*

This book, focused on the Sermon on the Mount, represents the second half of Mike and Rami's dialogue. In it, Mike and Rami explore the text of Jesus' sermon cooperatively, contributing perspectives drawn from their lives and religious traditions and seeking moments of illumination.

978-1-57312-654-0  254 pages/pb  **$19.00**

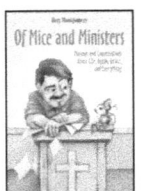
### Of Mice and Ministers
Musings and Conversations About Life, Death, Grace, and Everything
*Bert Montgomery*

With stories about pains, joys, and everyday life, *Of Mice and Ministers* finds Jesus in some unlikely places and challenges us to do the same. From tattooed women ministers to saying the "N"-word to the brotherly kiss, Bert Montgomery takes seriously the lesson from Psalm 139—where can one go that God is not already there?
978-1-57312-733-2  154 pages/pb  **$14.00**

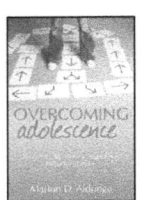
### Overcoming Adolescence
Growing Beyond Childhood into Maturity
*Marion D. Aldridge*

In *Overcoming Adolescence*, Marion D. Aldridge poses questions for adults of all ages to consider. His challenge to readers is one he has personally worked to confront: to grow up *all the way*—mentally, physically, academically, socially, emotionally, and spiritually. The key involves not only knowing how to work through the process but also how to recognize what may be contributing to our perpetual adolescence.
978-1-57312-577-2  156 pages/pb  **$17.00**

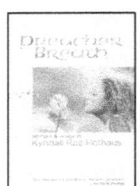
### Preacher Breath
Sermon & Essays
*Kyndall Rae Rothaus*

"The task of preaching is such an oddly wonderful, strangely beautiful experience. . . . Kyndall Rothaus's *Preacher Breath* is a worthy guide, leading the reader room by room with wisdom, depth, and a spiritual maturity far beyond her years, so that the preaching house becomes a holy, joyful home. . . . This book is soul kindle for a preacher's heart."
—Danielle Shroyer
Pastor and Author of *The Boundary-Breaking God*
978-1-57312-734-9  208 pages/pb  **$16.00**

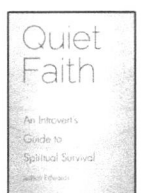
### Quiet Faith
An Introvert's Guide to Spiritual Survival
*Judson Edwards*

In eight finely crafted chapters, Edwards looks at key issues like evangelism, interpreting the Bible, dealing with doubt, and surviving the church from the perspective of a confirmed, but sometimes reluctant, introvert. In the process, he offers some provocative insights that introverts will find helpful and reassuring.
978-1-57312-681-6  144 pages/pb  **$15.00**

To order call **1-800-747-3016** or visit **www.helwys.com**

### Reading Deuteronomy
### (Reading the Old Testament series)
A Literary and Theological Commentary
*Stephen L. Cook*

A lost treasure for large segments of the modern world, the book of Deuteronomy powerfully repays contemporary readers' attention. God's presence and Word in Deuteronomy stir deep longing for God and move readers to a place of intimacy with divine otherness, holism, and will for person-centered community. The consistently theological interpretation reveals the centrality of Deuteronomy for faith and counters critical accusations about violence, intolerance, and polytheism in the book.   *978-1-57312-757-8  286 pages/pb*  **$22.00**

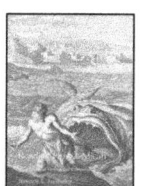

### Reading Hosea–Micah
### (Reading the Old Testament series)
A Literary and Theological Commentary
*Terence E. Fretheim*

Terence E. Fretheim explores themes of indictment, judgment, and salvation in Hosea–Micah. The indictment against the people of God especially involves issues of idolatry, as well as abuse of the poor and needy. The effects of such behaviors are often horrendous in their severity. While God is often the subject of such judgments, the consequences, like fruit, grow out of the deed itself.   *978-1-57312-687-8  224 pages/pb*  **$22.00**

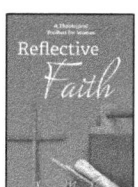

### Reflective Faith
A Theological Toolbox for Women
*Tony W. Cartledge*

In *Reflective Faith*, Susan Shaw offers a set of tools to explore difficult issues of biblical interpretation, theology, church history, and ethics—especially as they relate to women. Reflective faith invites intellectual struggle and embraces the unknown; it is a way of discipleship, a way to love God with your mind, as well as your heart, your soul, and your strength.
*978-1-57312-719-6  292 pages/pb*  **$24.00**
*Workbook 978-1-57312-754-7  164 pages/pb*  **$12.00**

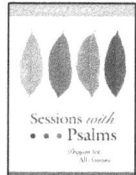

### Sessions with Psalms (Session Bible Studies series)
Prayers for All Seasons
*Eric and Alicia D. Porterfield*

Sessions with Psalms is a ten-session study unit designed to explore what it looks like for the words of the psalms to become the words of our prayers. Each session is followed by a thought-provoking page of questions that allow for a deeper experience of the scriptural passages. These resource pages can be used by seminar leaders during preparation and group discussion, as well as in individual Bible study.   *978-1-57312-768-4  136 pages/pb*  **$14.00**

**To order call 1-800-747-3016 or visit www.helwys.com**

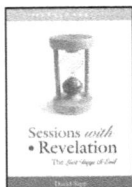

### Sessions with Revelation (Session Bible Studies series)
The Final Days of Evil

*David Sapp*

David Sapp's careful guide through Revelation demonstrates that it is a letter of hope for believers; it is less about the last days of history than it is about the last days of evil. Without eliminating its mystery, Sapp unlocks Revelation's central truths so that its relevance becomes clear.  978-1-57312-706-6  166 pages/pb  **$14.00**

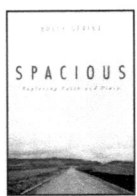

### Spacious
Exploring Faith and Place

*Holly Sprink*

Exploring where we are and why that matters to God is an ongoing process. If we are present and attentive, God creatively and continuously widens our view of the world.  978-1-57312-649-6  156 pages/pb  **$16.00**

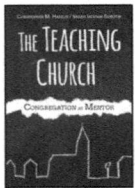

### The Teaching Church
Congregation as Mentor

*Christopher M. Hamlin / Sarah Jackson Shelton*

Collected in *The Teaching Church: Congregation as Mentor* are the stories of the pastors who shared how congregations have shaped, nurtured, and, sometimes, broken their resolve to be faithful servants of God.  978-1-57312-682-3  112 pages/pb  **$13.00**

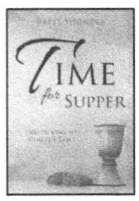

### Time for Supper
Invitations to Christ's Table

*Brett Younger*

Some scholars suggest that every meal in literature is a communion scene. Could every meal in the Bible be a communion text? Could every passage be an invitation to God's grace? At the Lord's Table we experience sorrow, hope, friendship, and forgiveness. These meditations on the Lord's Supper help us listen to the myriad of ways God invites us to gratefully, reverently, and joyfully share the cup of Christ.  978-1-57312-720-2  246 pages/pb  **$18.00**

To order call **1-800-747-3016** or visit **www.helwys.com**

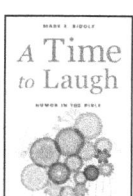

### A Time to Laugh
Humor in the Bible

*Mark E. Biddle*

An extension of his well-loved seminary course on humor in the Bible, A Time to Laugh draws on Mark E. Biddle's command of Hebrew language and cultural subtleties to explore the ways humor was intentionally incorporated into Scripture. With characteristic liveliness, Biddle guides the reader through the stories of six biblical characters who did rather unexpected things.  *978-1-57312-683-0   164 pages/pb*  **$14.00**

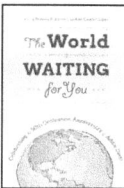

### The World Is Waiting for You
Celebrating the 50th Ordination Anniversary of Addie Davis

*Pamela R. Durso & LeAnn Gunter Johns, eds.*

Hope for the church and the world is alive and well in the words of these gifted women. Keen insight, delightful observations, profound courage, and a gift for communicating the good news are woven throughout these sermons. The Spirit so evident in Addie's calling clearly continues in her legacy.  *978-1-57312-732-5   224 pages/pb*  **$18.00**

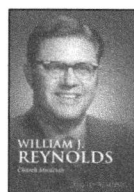

### William J. Reynolds
Church Musician

*David W. Music*

William J. Reynolds is renowned among Baptist musicians, music ministers, song leaders, and hymnody students. In eminently readable style, David W. Music's comprehensive biography describes Reynolds's family and educational background, his career as a minister of music, denominational leader, and seminary professor.  *978-1-57312-690-8   358 pages/pb*  **$23.00**

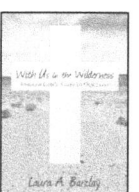

### With Us in the Wilderness
Finding God's Story in Our Lives

*Laura A. Barclay*

What stories compose your spiritual biography? In *With Us in the Wilderness*, Laura Barclay shares her own stories of the intersection of the divine and the everyday, guiding readers toward identifying and embracing God's presence in their own narratives.
*978-1-57312-721-9   120 pages/pb*  **$13.00**

---

To order call **1-800-747-3016** or visit **www.helwys.com**

# Clarence Jordan's
# Cotton Patch Gospel

## The Complete Collection

Hardback • 448 pages
Retail 50.00 • Your Price 25.00

Paperback • 448 pages
Retail 40.00 • Your Price 20.00

*The Cotton Patch Gospel,* by Koinonia Farm founder Clarence Jordan, recasts the stories of Jesus and the letters of the New Testament into the language and culture of the mid-twentieth-century South. Born out of the civil rights struggle, these now-classic translations of much of the New Testament bring the far-away places of Scripture closer to home: Gainesville, Selma, Birmingham, Atlanta, Washington D.C.

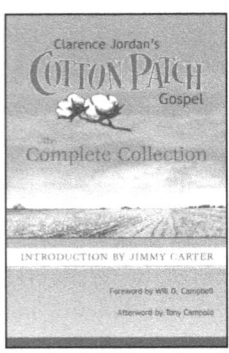

More than a translation, *The Cotton Patch Gospel* continues to make clear the startling relevance of Scripture for today. Now for the first time collected in a single, hardcover volume, this edition comes complete with a new Introduction by President Jimmy Carter, a Foreword by Will D. Campbell, and an Afterword by Tony Campolo. Smyth & Helwys Publishing is proud to help reintroduce these seminal works of Clarence Jordan to a new generation of believers, in an edition that can be passed down to generations still to come.

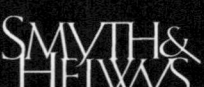 To order call **1-800-747-3016**
or visit **www.helwys.com**

www.ingramcontent.com/pod-product-compliance
Lightning Source LLC
Chambersburg PA
CBHW070540090426
42735CB00013B/3035